Sous Vide Master

Getting Started With Vacuum-Sealed Cooking, Delicious Recipes For Easy Cooking At Home, Modern Techniques for Perfect Cooking Through Science, Ultimate Low-Temperature Immersion Circulator Guide

Sarah P. Williamson

Sous Vide Master: Getting Started With Vacuum-Sealed Cooking, Delicious Recipes For Easy Cooking At Home, Modern Techniques for Perfect Cooking Through Science, Ultimate Low-Temperature Immersion Circulator Guide

Table of Contents

Book 1 - Sous Vide

Getting Started With Vacuum-Sealed Cooking (Authoritative Guide, Perfectly Cooked, Easy Gourmet At Home)

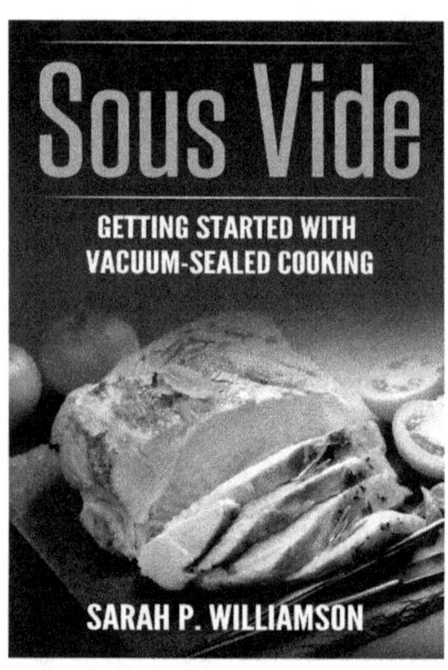

1 - Introduction

I want to thank you and congratulate you for buying this book.

Sous vide cooking is a simple and foolproof technique that ensures that you get tastier and more nutritious food. Even better, once you've gotten the process down, you are assured of getting the same great results every time you cook.

This book will teach you all the techniques you need to know in order to successfully cook sous vide, even without any fancy gadgets. We also provide you with a selection of recipes that you can try out once you've started cooking sous vide, so you can treat your family to some great dishes.

Thanks again for buying this book, I hope you enjoy it!

2 - What is Sous Vide?

Sous vide is French for "under vacuum" and refers to a culinary technique in which food is vacuum sealed and cooked while submerged in water that has been heated to a very precise and consistent temperature. Once the food hits the desired cooking temperature or time, it is taken out and served. Although it can be used to cook a variety of food, sous vide is most useful in cooking seafood and meat.

In conventional methods, food has to be cooked at a temperature high enough that its internal temperature reaches the level required to cook it. However, the risk is that the food would become overcooked when left at this temperature too long, turning it dry or burning it. Conversely, if the food is taken from the heat too early, the center may still be raw even if the outside is already cooked.

Sous vide addresses this problem by immersing the food in a water bath where the temperature of the water is set at the exact temperature required to ensure that its internal temperature reaches cooking level. This means that even if you leave the food immersed for a longer time than absolutely necessary, it does not overcook since its internal temperature cannot exceed the water temperature.

Sous vide had previously been mainly practiced by professional chefs since the equipment needed was expensive. In recent years, however, the prices have gone down, allowing home cooks to start trying sous vide cooking at home.

History of Sous Vide

The basic idea of cooking food packaged in airtight containers was actually first conceived in the eighteenth century by inventor Sir Benjamin Thompson, although the heat transfer medium was air rather than water. But it was never more than a theory to him, and Thompson never developed a dedicated machine to put his ideas to practical use.

However, the basic idea was later developed as a method of food preservation, with food being vacuum-sealed in jars, and then boiled to kill harmful bacteria and other contaminants like yeasts. As long as the seal remained unbroken, the food inside would remain unspoiled.

In the 1960s, cryovacking or vacuum sealing food under pressure in food-grade plastic pouches and film was developed. This paved the way for modern sous vide.

In 1974, Chef George Pralus, who was working at the Michelin three-star rated La Maison Troisgros, was looking for a method of cooking delicate fois gras that reduced wastage. When fois gras was cooked using traditional methods, it shrank to nearly half its size, which cost the restaurant a lot of money.

Pralus had heard about the vacuum-packing method being used to preserve foods so he decided to try applying it to food preparation. He wrapped the fois gras in multiple layers of plastic to create a vacuum and then submerged it in a water bath to cook it. The experiment was successful and sous vide, as we know it today, was born.

While Pralus was developing sous vide as a cooking technique, Bruno Goussalt was experimenting with it as a way of preserving food on a large scale. His experiments paved the way for sous vide companies that made classical dishes for restaurants that only needed to be reheated to serve.

Since Goussalt's methods focused on food preservation, they paved the way for sous vide to be used professionally since they allowed it to meet French standards for food safety.

However, sous vide was initially mainly used by professional chefs over the next few decades. This method of cooking was still considered mostly experimental and potentially dangerous if not done properly. Also, the equipment used for sous vide cooking was made for commercial kitchens, costing thousands of dollars, and thus was too expensive for most households.

But in the 2000s, books about sous vide, such as chef Thomas Keller's Under Pressure: Cooking Sous Vide, were becoming popular, sparking interest in technique among serious home chefs.

Since affordable equipment was not available to them, they experimented with homemade kits using sealable bags and kettles. Although these were successful to some degree, it was only when smaller sous vide equipment specifically designed for home use began being produced that the technique really achieved its current popularity.

Basic Features of Sous Vide Cooking

The food to be cooked is vacuum-sealed in a plastic bag. This seals in the aroma and juices of the food that may be lost during the cooking process.

The bag is immersed in a water bath that is heated to the exact cooking temperature. This ensures the food cannot be overcooked since the temperature of the food cannot exceed that of the water in the bath. In traditional cooking methods, the temperature must be set higher than the final desired cook temperature and the food must be removed from the heat to avoid overcooking.

The vacuum inside the bag allows the cooked food to be stored for a longer period of time as long as it is placed immediately in the refrigerator while still sealed.

You no longer need to time your cooking so precisely. In traditional cooking methods, food is cooked at a high temperature that fluctuates, so you have to time it precisely. If you leave the food on the flame for just a few minutes too long, the food may be overcooked or not taste as good.

On the other hand, with sous vide, there is a higher margin of error; even if you overcook for just a few minutes, the food will still taste as good.

Benefits of Sous Vide Cooking

Since sous vide allows you to cook food for longer periods at lower temperatures, it allows you to enjoy many benefits, including:

Tastier food since sous-vide cooking means it does not lose its original aroma, flavor, weight and natural color since it cooks at a lower temperature. Food also does not lose its form or dehydrate while cooking.

Since food cooked sous-vide maintains enhanced flavor, you don't need additional fat or salt to taste; the food also retains its nutrients while cooking.

You can get more consistent results when you cook since precise temperatures are used during cooking.

You have more control over the timing of your cooking. By setting the water bath at the right temperature, you can cook the food more slowly so that it will be ready by the time you get home. You can even set it to cook overnight so that it will be done when you get up in the morning.

Cooking meals sous-vide is quick and easy. Once you've prepared the food, all you have to do is place it in the pre-heated water bath. You can be done in as little as thirty minutes.

You can place individual servings in their own bags, allowing you to easily cook large quantities for dinner parties and other get-togethers.

Since you can cook smaller portions, there is less food wastage, saving you money. Many sous vide water baths also use less energy than traditional electric or gas ovens.

Food cooked sous vide lasts longer. You can prepare food in advance, then freeze it after cooling, and thaw it for later.

3 - Sous Vide Equipment: What You Need

One of the best things about sous vide cooking is that you can choose your equipment based on your budget. If you have the money to spend, you can buy sous vide water baths with temperature controls.

But if you are just starting out and have limited funds, you can buy a more affordable immersion circulator that ensures heat is evenly distributed throughout the water but does not have its own dedicated water container.

Although specialized sous vide machines are more expensive, they allow you to start cooking at once and are basically foolproof; all you have to do is fill the container with water, set the temperature and place the bags with the food you're cooking into the bath. In addition, these machines generate higher temperatures and are insulated to ensure that the cooking temperature remains at an even level.

When choosing one of these machines, one of the main considerations is the capacity of the water bath. Generally, the machines available have capacities that range from a low of five liters to as much as 120 liters.

A machine with a larger capacity gives you more flexibility to cook the quantities that you need, but of course will be bulkier and more difficult to store if you have limited counter space. Also, when deciding on the capacity, keep in mind that you should fill only half the bath with pouches since there needs to be room to allow the water to circulate.

Other considerations to keep in mind are their ability to keep the temperature stable and its heating power, which determines how long it takes to reach the required temperature. Some models also come with a vacuum sealer that makes it more convenient to use since you can easily ensure that there is no air in the bag before you place it in the water bath.

Immersion circulators are essentially heating wands that are placed into a water container; they will heat the water and keep it at a consistent temperature. They can heat up to five gallons of water, providing you with plenty of flexibility for cooking.

The main disadvantage of using these machines is that, since they are used in open containers, there are issues with water evaporation and heat loss. But you can address this issue by using a polycarbonate container with a lid and then cutting a hole in the lid to accommodate the circulator. An inexpensive plastic cooler also works very well since it is insulated which will help maintain the temperature.

Alternately, you can cover the opening of the container with aluminum foil or plastic wrap to keep the heat in and reduce evaporation. However, they are not easy to remove and replace, which makes it difficult if you want to add water or adjust the food pouches.

The simplest and most effective solution, however, is to simply place Ping-Pong balls on top of the bath. A layer of these balls will condense steam so it drips back down and helps maintain the water level while keeping the water insulated. You can also easily place and remove food packets from the water bath and the balls will adjust to the shape of your water container; the balls are also reusable.

If you don't have the budget to purchase a circulator or stand-alone sous vide machine, however, it is possible to create a basic sous vide setup at home using basic materials such as a pot and a stove; however, you will need to invest in an instant-read digital thermometer if you don't have one. We will describe how in the following chapter.

4 - How to Cook Sous Vide

To give you a better understanding of how to cook sous-vide, here is a step-by-step overview of the process.

Determine the right temperature for the food you are planning to cook. This is one of the essential steps in cooking sous vide since the temperature of the water has to be as close as possible to the optimal temperature to get the best results.

For beginners, however, you can start by determining the temperature range for the 'done-ness' of the food you are cooking, i.e. medium-rare, medium, traditional, as well as the type of food, i.e. chicken or beef.

Preparing the food for cooking

There are a number of ways to prepare food before placing it in the bag, ranging from pre-portioning, slicing, blanching and smoking.

Package the food. Basically, this involves sealing the food to be cooked in plastic bags that you can remove the air from, such as food grade Ziploc bags. For some foods, however, glass jars can be an option.

Cook the food at the required time. Although sous vide is generally used for cooking, you can also use it to tenderize tough pieces of meat. Tenderizing means you will have to cook the meat for hours or even days, depending on how tender you want it to be.

Also, a consideration when deciding cooking times is food safety. Since the temperatures used in sous-vide are relatively low, you can only cook food for a limited amount of time. This range is from 40-degrees F to 140-degrees F, and food cooked at this temperature for longer than a few hours becomes unsafe.

Also, a consideration is the size of the piece you are cooking; if the piece is too big, the heat may not be enough to ensure that it is thoroughly cooked, leaving certain areas vulnerable to microbial spoilage.

Adding finishing touches

Since the temperatures used in sous vide cooking are too low to brown meat, you have to sear steaks after cooking to give them a crust and the expected flavor. However, you can sear meat before and after cooking to get better results.

5 - Basic Sous Vide Cooking

Before you invest in sous vide equipment, you might want to try cooking using the sous vide method first, so you can see how it works and what food cooked with this technique tastes like.

The basic method simply involves bagging some strips of food in a Ziploc bag and immersing them in hot water. Here are two simple recipes you can try; all you need is a deep kitchen sink that can accommodate several gallons of hot water or a five-gallon cooler that will keep in the heat.

The first recipe is for cooking salmon filet. This delicate fish is ideal to cook sous vide since it easily contracts and dries out when exposed to too much heat. Take some salmon strips and place one or more strips per bag, but make sure that they are in a single layer. Make sure that you remove most of the air (use the water displacement method described later in the chapter).

Add some olive oil or melted butter, and then fill your container with hot water that is around 122-degrees F; if you use your kitchen sink, you don't need to worry about excessive heat loss since large volumes of hot water will be able to retain its temperature. Immerse the bags in water for around fifteen minutes. Then remove the salmon from the water.

Once you've finished cooking the salmon, you can finish it before serving by searing it in a pan. First heat the pan until it is sizzling; test it by flicking some water drops onto it. Place a thin layer of oil on the pan (olive oil if you have it, otherwise canola oil will do). Place the filets on the pan with the skin side down, and let brown for thirty seconds to one minute.

You can also use this basic method for cooking steaks. Take a pair of strip steaks (less than ¼-inch) and season them. Bag them in a single layer, and then add some canola oil. Boil some water in a pot until it reaches 145-degrees F.

Fill the cooler or kitchen sink with water and immerse the bags; make sure they are completely immersed to ensure they will be fully cooked. Allow the steaks to cook for around an hour. Then remove from the water and serve as desired or finish by heating in a pan.

Since cooking times are more forgiving with sous vide, you don't have to worry about overcooking even if you leave the food in the hot water for longer than the recommended cooking time; just don't take them out too early since they may be under-cooked.

As we mentioned in the previous chapter, you can create a basic sous vide setup without having to invest in a standalone machine or immersion circulator. All you need is a pot and a digital instant-read thermometer. The biggest challenge with using this basic setup is maintaining the required cooking temperature long enough to cook the food.

Since pots can easily lose temperature through the sides, as well as through water evaporation, you will have to constantly adjust the heat on the stove to ensure that the temperature remains steady. Fortunately, you don't have to keep the temperature at an exact level, and losing a degree or two is not that big of a deal.

All you have to do to cook sous vide is to fill the pot with water up to a level that it will not overflow once you place the food bags inside. Then heat the water until it reaches the required temperature, using the digital thermometer to measure it.

This can take a bit of time and practice to get right; however, frequently stirring the water can help it reach the required temperature more quickly. To help you monitor the temperature, you can attach the digital thermometer on a binder clip or a skewer so you can mount it to the side of the pot.

Choosing Cooking Times and Temperatures

When you cook a piece of meat using traditional methods, one of the major issues you have to address is that the outside heats more quickly than the center. Thus, it becomes difficult to determine when the meat is completely done; a lot of times, the outside is already done while the center is still relatively uncooked.

With sous vide cooking, however, this discrepancy is easily addressed, allowing you to get a perfectly cooked piece of meat. Since you are cooking using a precise temperature that is maintained at a static level, you can more readily predict how long it will take the center to reach cooking temperature.

Once submerged in the water bath, the food will cook evenly all over, from edge to center, because the cooking temperature and the external temperatures are one and the same.

When determining how long to cook meat, the main consideration is the thickness of the meat; the thicker the meat, the longer it takes to cook. In addition, although sous vide is more forgiving when it comes to cooking times, there is still a maximum time beyond which you should not keep food in the water, otherwise it becomes mushy.

6 - Guide to choosing the right temperatures and times for cooking various food groups

Fish

Fish are cooked only for a short time and the result is moist and flaky. You can eat it as is with some lemon juice or olive oil or with a fresh vegetable salsa as a side dish, make it a sandwich or add it to traditional dishes such as fish chowder and fish stew.

Generally, depending on the level of doneness you want, fish is cooked at 104-degrees F (rare sushi); 122-degrees F (medium rare sushi); 132-degrees F (medium rare) and 140-degrees F (medium) for 10 to 30 minutes. For most cuts, however, setting your machine to 130-degrees F will be sufficient.

Chicken

Sous vide results in chicken that is very moist and uniformly tender, making it the ideal basis for dishes that use chicken with a coating, such as fried chicken and chicken parmigiana.

Generally, the chicken should be cooked at 147-degrees F for one to four hours (breast) and 4 to 8 hours (thighs or legs). Although you can cook chicken at less than 140-degrees F, it tastes raw.

Eggs can be cooked at a range of 135-degrees F (safe to eat but is 'raw') to 158-degrees F (very hard boiled), with the ideal at 148-degrees F, although you can experiment to find the right temperature. Some people may boil it for two to five minutes after cooking to solidify the egg while without overcooking the yolk.

Pork

Sous vide allows you to cook pork medium-rare while maintaining food safety, as well as tenderizing tougher cuts by cooking them for longer at temperatures low enough to avoid drying them out. According to FDA guidelines, pork is safe when cooked at 130-degrees F for more than 112 minutes and 140-degrees F for over 12 minutes.

Generally, when cooking pork you can set your machine to 131-degrees F (medium rare) for six to twelve hours or 140-degrees F (medium) for five to ten hours. For tougher cuts you can cook it at 155-degrees F: to get it well done. You can also cook frozen pork chops without having to defrost them first; just add an additional fifteen to twenty minutes cooking time. Cooking times for various cuts are as follows:

- Tenderloin: medium rare 3 to 6 hours/medium 2 to 4 hours

- Pork loin chop: medium rare 3 to 5 hours/medium 2 to 4 hours

- Pork loin roast: medium rare 4 to 8 hours/medium 4 to 6 hours

- Pork ribs chop/roast: medium rare 5 to 8 hours/medium 4 to 7 hours

- Pork sirloin chop/roast: medium rare 6 to 12 hours/medium 5 to 10 hours/well done 10 to 16 hours (roast)

- Ribs Back/Baby Back/Country Style: medium rare 8 to 12 hours/medium 8 to 12 hours/well 12 to 24 hours

- Spare Ribs: medium rare/rare/well 12 to 24 hours

- Fresh Ham (Pork Leg): medium rare/rare/well 10 to 20 hours

- Ground Pork: medium rare/rare 2 to 4 hours

- Pork Sausage: medium rare/rare/well 2 to 3 hours

- Pork Chops: medium rare 3 to 6 hours/medium 2 to 4 hours

- Pork Belly/Fresh Side: low 140-degrees F 2 to 3 days/in-between 160-degrees F 18 to 36 hours/high 180-degrees F 12 to 18 hours

Beef Roasts

Cooking tough cuts of beef sous vide allows you to tenderize them without drying them out since they never go beyond medium rare cooking temperatures. Generally, you can set your machine to 131-degrees F to 140-degrees F for most cuts, although you can set it to 160-degrees F if you want them to be well done. Cooking times are as follows:

- Prime Rib/ Sirloin/Tri-Tip Roast: medium rare/medium 5 to 10 hours

- Chuck Roast/Short Ribs: medium rare/medium 2 to 3 days, well 1 to 2 days

- Top Round Roast: medium rare/medium 1 to 3 days, well 1 to 2 days

- Bottom Round Roast/Brisket/Cheek/Shank/Pot Roast: medium rare/medium 2 to 3 days, well 1 to 2 days

- Beef Stew: medium rare/medium 4 to 8 hours

Beef Steaks

More tender cuts of beef are cooked at 131-degrees F to 140-degrees F and should not exceed this temperature since the beef will begin to dry out. Cooking times are generally between 2 to 4 hours, resulting in a more tender steak. You can cook tougher steaks for longer times, and they will be as tender as tenderloin.

Cooking times are:

- Tenderloin/Porterhouse/T-Bone/Top Loin Strip: medium rare/medium 2 to 3 hours

- Ribeye/Rib: medium rare/medium 2 to 8 hours

- Tri-Tip/Sirloin: medium rare/medium 2 to 10 hours

- Flat Iron/Shoulder/Blade: medium rare/medium 4 to 10 hours

- Chuck/Eye Round/Top Round/Skirt/Flank: medium rare/medium 1 to 2 days

- Hamburger: medium rare/medium 2 to 4 hours

Turkey

Cooking turkey sous vide results in meat that is very moist and uniformly tender. Generally, turkey should be cooked at temperatures above 140-degrees F, with the ideal cooking temperature at 136-degrees F (rare) or 147-degrees F (medium) at 1 to 4 hours for breasts and 148-degrees F (ideal) for 4 to 8 hours for thighs, drumsticks, and legs; if you want the latter at medium-rare doneness, cook the latter at 140-degrees F for 3 to 4 hours and at 160-degrees F for 18 to 24 hours if they are going to be shredded. You can also use the juices in the bag as gravy to serve the turkey with.

However, you should remove the skin before cooking because it will not become crisp; you can crisp it before serving by frying it in a skillet with a little oil or bake it in the oven at 375-degrees F on a baking sheet with raised edges to catch the fat.

Duck

Cooking duck sous vide allows you to consistently get outstanding results but also easily confit duck. Duck is generally cooked at 131-degrees F to medium rate doneness and for 2 to 4 hours. If you are planning to cook duck for shredding, you should cook it at 176-degrees F to well doneness and for 8 to 10 hours; the duck will still be moist but will be fall apart ready for shredding. To make duck confit, all you have to do is prepare the meat by curing it and then bag it with some duck fat; cook for 10 to 20 hours at 167-degrees F.

As with other poultry meats such as chicken and turkey, you should remove the skin before putting it in the bag and crisp it separately.

Shellfish

Cooking this seafood sous vide lets you avoid the pitfalls of cooking it the traditional way, which is that it becomes tough, and gives you very tender results. Although the ideal cooking temperature is 132-degrees F, shellfish will not be pasteurized and you should avoid it if you have a susceptible immune system or the shellfish is sushi-grade.

Cooking times and temperatures are as follows:

- Lobster: cooking time 15 to 40 minutes medium rare 126-degrees F/medium 140-degrees F

- Shrimp: cooking time 15 to 35 minutes medium rare (sushi) 122-degrees F/medium rare 132-degrees F

- Squid: pre-sear 45 minutes to 1 hour at 113-degrees F/low heat 2 to 4 hours at 138-degrees F/high heat 60 minutes at 180-degrees F

- Soft shell crab: 3 hours at 145-degrees F to 150-degrees F

- Scallops: pre-sear 15 to 35 minutes at 122-degrees F

- Octopus: slow 4 to 7 hours at 170-degrees F/fast 2 to 3 hours at 180-degrees F

Lamb

Sous vide is the perfect method for cooking this meat due to its toughness. By cooking it at lower temperatures for a longer period, you can tenderize the meat without drying it out. Tough cuts of lamb are generally cooked for one to two days to fully tenderize although tenderer roasts will be fully tenderized at 2 to 4 hours.

Lamb is generally cooked for 2 to 3 hours at 131-degrees F to get medium-rare doneness, for 1 to 3 hours at 140-degrees F to get medium doneness or for 1 to 2 hours at 126-degrees F to get rare doneness. However, you should exercise care since lamb cooked at less than 130-degrees F is still not pasteurized and may not be safe to eat if you have a sensitive immune system.

Cooking instructions for lamb:

- Lamb leg, boneless: cooking time 18 to 36 hours medium rare at 131-degrees F/medium at 140-degrees F

- Lamb leg, bone-in: medium rare 2 to 3 days at 131-degrees F/medium 1 to 3 days at 140-degrees F

- Shank/Shoulder: medium rare 1 to 2 days at 131-degrees F/medium 1 to 2 days at 140-degrees F/well 165-degrees F 18 to 36 hours (shoulder) 1 to 2 days (shank)

- Breast: cooking time 20 to 28 hours medium-rare 131-degrees F/medium 140-degrees F/well 165-degrees F

- Ribs: cooking time 22 to 26 hours medium-rare 131-degrees F/medium 140-degrees F/well 165-degrees F

- Osso Buco: cooking time 1 to 2 days medium-rare 131-degrees F/medium 140-degrees F/well 165-degrees F

Fruits and vegetables

By cooking these foods sous vide you can preserve their nutrients and tenderize them without risking them becoming too soft and losing their structure. In addition, any nutrients that drip out of vegetables will be caught in the bag so they can be reused.

When cooking fruits and vegetables sous vide, set the machine to 183-degrees F. Cooking times will vary depending on their firmness. The cooking times for selected fruits and vegetables are:

- Broccoli: 20 to 30 minutes

- Brussels Sprouts: 45 to 60 minutes

- Cabbage: 30 to 45 minutes

- Cauliflower: 20 to 30 minutes/puree 2 hours

- Zucchini: 30 to 60 minutes

- Pumpkin: 45 to 60 minutes

- Leek: 30 to 60 minutes

- Onion: 35 to 45 minutes

- Green Beans: 30 to 45 minutes

- Corn: 30 to 45 minutes

- Pea Pods: 30 to 40 minutes

- Beet: 30 minutes to 1 hour

- Carrot: 40 minutes to 1 hour

- Turnip: 30 to 45 minutes

- Potatoes: small 30 minutes to 1 hour/large 1 to 2 hours

- Sweet potatoes: small 45 minutes to 1 hour/large 1 hour to 90 minutes

- Artichokes: 45 to 75 minutes

- Asparagus: 30 to 40 minutes

- Apple: 25 to 40 minutes

- Pears: 25 to 35 minutes

- Banana: 10 to 15 minutes

- Cherries: 15 to 25 minutes

- Pineapple: 45 minutes to 1 hour

- Plums: 15 to 20 minutes

- Peaches: 30 minutes to 1 hour

- Eggplant: 30 to 45 minutes

- Garlic: 1 hour to 90 minutes

7 - Preparing Food for Sous Vide Cooking

The basic way to prepare food for sous vide is to slice or pre-portion it. This is recommended for delicate cuts of meat and fish since it would lessen the cooking time and ensure that the food does not become mushy.

Smaller portions mean the center of the meat or fish reaches final cooking temperature more quickly. It also ensures food safety since every part of the piece reaches cooking temperature. However, tougher cuts of meat can be cooked in larger pieces since you get better results with longer cooking times.

Searing meat

If you are cooking steak and other meats, they will not achieve the crispy and flavorful skin that gives them most of their flavor when cooking sous vide due to the low temperatures used. Hence, meat has to be seared before cooking, although there are some who prefer to do it afterward.

Searing beforehand has several benefits, including reducing the chances of overcooking and ensuring better flavor since the flavor compounds penetrate the meat during cooking.

In addition, you ensure better food safety since pre-searing kills most of the germs that can cause the meat to go bad.

However, the crust will be softened during the cooking process, and to restore it, you will have to sear the meat again before serving. But pre-searing means the process will be quicker.

In addition, pre-searing is not recommended for the meat of lamb and other grass-fed animals, since it can result in unpleasant flavors when cooking sous vide for a long time.

Before searing meat, you will have to dry it out since a moist surface will prevent browning, forcing you to cook it for longer and risking overcooking. Once you take it out of the packet, pat it dry with clean towels or paper towels.

Dry it a few minutes before searing so that the meat will cool slightly and any moisture left behind will evaporate. However, if you would like to get a deeper crust, you can cool the meat for longer, since this will give you more time to brown it before you risk overcooking.

There are a number of ways you can sear meat. The easiest method is to sear it in a pan, which is particularly effective if you have a cast-iron skillet; if you are planning to sear fish or other delicate seafood, however, a stainless steel pan should be used.

All you have to do is place a thin layer of refined oil with a high smoke point (i.e. canola oil) on the skillet and heat it over medium or high heat until it starts to smoke and turns brown, and then cook the food for 45 to 90 seconds per side until it browns.

Alternately, you can deep fry food to brown it. Use a pan filled with oil just below the halfway level that has been heated to 375-degrees – 400-degrees F. Place the food in the oil and fry for 30 to 90 seconds.

For roasts, you can use an oven. Coat the roast with your desired coating after sous vide cooking, and then cook it in an oven set to 500-degrees F. You can also use a grill, whether gas-fired or coal.

Make sure the heat is turned all the way up or the coals are as hot as possible and let the bars fully heat after closing the lid. Brush the meat with some oil and place on the grill with the lid open; cook for 45 to 90 seconds, until grill marks form and the meat is browned.

Finally, you can use a torch, which is particularly effective for foods that have an uneven surface. If you are planning to invest in a torch for searing, you will have to buy a larger one that is suited for industrial uses such as light welding and soldering copper, and which produces temperatures of more than 3500-degrees F, which is enough to sear food in 2 to 3 minutes.

Although there are a wide variety of torches available on the market, the most reliable ones seem to be those produced by BernzOmatic, which has been in existence for over a century.

The most affordable torches are those that use propane gas, although some may prefer MAP-Pro, even though it carries a price premium. When searing, make sure that the torch is producing the fully oxidizing flame, which is dark blue, relatively short and produces a hissing sound.

If you sear food using a large yellow flame, you may end up producing food with 'torch taste', which is unpleasant. Point the torch at the food and make sure to keep it moving to avoid uneven browning.

Blanching vegetables

You can cook vegetables sous vide by placing entire pieces

into the bag and then slicing them after they're done. However, you should blanch them before cooking to preserve their texture and color. Simply immerse the vegetables in boiling water for two seconds to destroy the enzymes that cause browning.

Seasoning food

If you would like to add dry or wet condiments to food before cooking, use smaller quantities than you would normally since the flavors will be more intense. You will also have to vacuum pack the food.

To ensure that liquid condiments are not sucked into the machine when vacuum packing, freeze them beforehand; however, this will not be necessary if you are using a vacuum chamber since it can handle liquids easily.

Sealing Food for Sous Vide

When sealing food inside the bag for sous vide, you don't actually need to create a vacuum seal for the process to work; you only need to make sure that most of the air inside the bag is removed. This ensures that flavors are sealed in and not lost to the water; bags that have air in them also float, which means that some of the food may not be cooked since it is out of the water.

The most common containers used to package food for sous vide cooking are sealable plastic bags. Use food-grade polyethylene, polypropylene or low-density polyethylene bags.

You can use specially made sous vide bags or high-quality Ziploc bags (gallon freezer bags will be big enough to accommodate several servings at once). However, if you're planning to cook food above 158-degrees F, you should use sous vide bags rather than Ziploc bags, since the seams of the latter may fail; if you don't have any sous vide bags, you can improvise by double bagging Ziploc bags.

Vacuum sealers are not necessary to cook sous vide since the seals of Ziploc or sous vide bags are secure enough. However, if you plan to cook a lot of vegetables, you might want to invest in an inexpensive sealer in order to be assured of the best results. You can also use the sealer to store food so that they will keep longer by removing the air inside the bag.

Even without a vacuum sealer, however, there is a simple way to ensure that air is removed from your sous vide bags.

7 - PREPARING FOOD FOR SOUS VIDE COOKING

1. Fill a bowl or your kitchen sink with water.

2. Place ingredients in Ziploc bag up to an inch from the mouth, then close the seal with only a small opening left.

3. Slowly submerge the bag in the water until the open mouth is left exposed. This will force all the air out.

4. Zip the opening closed.

What about canning jars as an alternative? Some people prefer glass jars for sous vide due to concerns about the safety of plastic, even though Ziploc bags are perfectly safe since they only soften at 195-degrees F that is lower than most temperatures used in sous vide. Although they work fine, it will take longer for your food to cook.

In addition, when cooking meat you will have to cover it with a cooking liquid such as oil to ensure that it is cooked safely. However, jars are recommended if you are batch-cooking yogurt, custard or other foods that need to set; you can distribute portions among the small jars and then cook them.

8 - Tips for Successful Sous Vide Cooking

Don't let the water in the bath evaporate

If the water level falls below the heating coils of the sous vide machine or circulator motor, it can cause damage to the unit you are using. This is a particular issue if you are cooking for an extended period of time. So make sure that your water bath is covered with a lid, plastic wrap or layer of Ping-Pong balls.

Choose the seasonings and herbs you use carefully

Fresh herbs such as onions and garlic don't seem to do as well during sous vide cooking as dried ones such as black pepper and cumin. If left too long, these herbs may even overpower the flavor of the food and even eventually taste rancid.

Make sure that the bags are completely immersed in the hot water

If you have successfully removed all the air from the bag,

this should not be a problem unless the food item you are cooking is lightweight. In this case, you can add a food-safe weight to the bag, such as a stainless steel dull butter knife, a clean glass marble or other stainless steel items. To avoid contamination, put these in their own smaller pouch before placing them in the food bag.

If the issue is that the bags are moving up and down because of the immersion circulator's motor, you can help keep the bags in place by using binder clips to attach them to the side of the water bath.

Avoid keeping meat in the water bath for longer than 72 hours

To avoid food safety issues, you should not cook meat sous vide for longer than three days. Botulism can easily develop in food that has been kept in a vacuum for too long since the bacteria which produces it needs an environment without air to grow. In addition, you should eat it as soon as possible after cooking.

Longer is not necessarily better

Although sous vide cooking is more forgiving in terms of the timing, you should still not keep food in the water bath for too long after the recommended time. The longer you keep meat in the sous vide bath, the more moisture it loses. Thus, no matter how long the recommended cooking time, a good rule of thumb to follow is that the meat should not be cooked longer than 36 hours.

If you are ready to cook sous vide seriously, here are some simple recipes that can get you started. Remember to read the recipe thoroughly before starting out, and prepare all the ingredients necessary before you begin cooking.

However, you should not hesitate to adjust quantities of ingredients based on your requirements, since these will not affect cooking times and temperatures too much. Once you've completed the recipe once, you can start experimenting by substituting some ingredients based on your preferences, in order to make a dish that is uniquely your own.

9 - Recipes

Sous Vide Pork Chops

One disadvantage of trying to eat healthier by using leaner cuts of pork is that these tend to dry out more quickly at high temperatures. Cooking them sous vide solves this problem since they are cooked at a lower temperature, resulting in juicier pork that is thoroughly cooked.

Depending on the level of doneness you want, you can set the temperature to 130-degrees F (rare), 140-degrees F (medium-rare), 150-degrees F (medium-well) and 160-degrees F (well done). Make sure the water has reached this final temperature before you place the pork chops in it.

If you are planning to cook the chops at once, generously season them using salt and pepper. If you are planning to leave them in the bag for more than a few hours before you cook them, season them only before you sear them after cooking.

To ensure that the juices of the pork will not get on the edge of the bag and interfere with the integrity of the seal, form a hem by folding the top back over itself. Slide the chops into a bag in one layer. Make sure that the bag is not too full; you can use several bags if necessary. Most of the air in the bag should be removed when sealing and the bag should sink when placed in the water.

Cooking time is determined by the thickness of the chops. For every half-inch thickness, allow fifteen minutes cooking time plus another ten as a margin of error.

Thus, if you have a steak that is 1-1/2 inches thick, you should cook it for at least an hour but no more than 4 hours; if you have thicker chops, then add another fifteen minutes per half-inch thickness. Don't let the pork stay in the water longer than four hours since the meat will become too tender and mushy.

After the pork is removed from the water, dry thoroughly with paper towels or kitchen towels. Place a skillet on the stove over high heat and then add one tablespoon of canola or vegetable oil and one tablespoon of butter. Swirl the pan until the butter starts to brown and is melting.

Put the pork on the skillet and cook for 45 seconds until crust is very crisp and deep brown. Flip and cook on the other side. Once they are browned, pick up the chops with tongs and brown the edges.

Place the chops on a rack set over a baking sheet for a couple of minutes and then serve. If you are not going to serve the chops at once, you can reheat the drippings until they sizzle, and then pour them over the chops to make the crust crisp again.

Sous Vide Fried Chicken Wings

This fried chicken recipe is healthier than traditional ones since it ensures that the wings are thoroughly cooked before they are fried, and you only have to fry them for a shorter time. This recipe is intended to serve four people but you can adjust it for greater or lesser servings.

Ingredients:

- Chicken wings, 8 pieces (dark or light meat)

- Soymilk, 2 cups

- Lemon juice or vinegar, one tablespoon

- Plain flour, one cup

- Rice flour, one cup

- Cornstarch or corn flour, half-cup

- Paprika, 2 tablespoons

- Salt 2 tablespoons

- Ground black pepper, 2 tablespoons

Procedure:

1. Heat water to a final temperature of 154.4-degrees F.

2. Season chicken with salt and pepper then bag it.

3. If dark meat, cook for 3 hours; if light, one hour.

Finishing

1. Remove chicken from water, dry thoroughly and set aside for fifteen to twenty minutes.

2. Preheat the oil in the fryer to 400-degrees F to 425-degrees F.

3. In a bowl, whisk together soy milk and vinegar or lemon juice. In another bowl, whisk together the dry ingredients.

4. Dredge the chicken in the dry and then the wet mixture. Repeat two to three times then place wings on a wire rack.

5. Deep fry chicken in batches of 2 to 3 pieces for three to four minutes. Set the fried pieces on a wire rack and let cool for fifteen to twenty minutes before serving.

Sous Vide Soft Poached Eggs

Eggs are among the easiest foods to cook sous vide since you don't even need a sous vide machine or a circulator. In this recipe we will include instructions on how you can cook poached eggs using only a large cooler; you can cook up to twelve eggs.

Procedure:

1. If you have a circulator or sous vide machine, set the temperature to 143-degrees F. If you are using a cooler, fill it with hot water; boil water in a kettle and pour it into the cooler to raise the temperature to 146-degrees F.

2. Place the eggs in the water bath and cook for forty-five minutes. Remove eggs from water and let cool for a while.

3. Fill a medium pot with water and bring it to a bare

simmer; then lower the heat until the water stops bubbling entirely.

4. Take one egg and gently crack it at the fat end; peel off a square opening around 1-1/2 inches. Invert egg over a small bowl and let slip out of the opening; if it has been cooked properly it will slip right out of the shell. Repeat with remaining eggs, using a separate bowl for each egg.

5. Carefully pick up eggs one at a time with a perforated spoon; dump excess whites and return eggs to bowls.

6. After all the eggs have been drained, slip them into the pot. Swirl the water occasionally so eggs won't stick to the bottom.

7. Cook for around a minute or until the white outside is just set. Use a perforated spoon to pick up eggs and serve immediately.

8. You can also keep the eggs in the refrigerator for as long as three days; just immerse them in cold water in a sealed container. Reheat eggs by placing them in a bowl with hot water for a few minutes.

Sous Vide Soft Boiled Eggs

You can also use a similar method to cook soft-boiled eggs. This recipe uses an ice bath to stop the cooking process and prepare the eggs for sous vide.

Procedure:

1. If you have a circulator or sous vide machine, set the temperature to 143-degrees F. If you are using a cooler, fill it with hot water; boil water in a kettle and pour it into the cooler to raise the temperature to 146-degrees F.

2. Prepare an ice bath by taking a metal container and filling it with cold water and ice.

3. Fill a large pot with water and bring it to high heat. Place eggs in a strainer or mesh spider and cook for precisely three minutes.

4. Transfer eggs immediately to the ice bath and let chill for a minute.

5. Let eggs cook in sous vide cooker or cooler for forty-five minutes.

6. Serve immediately.

7. You can also store the eggs in the refrigerator for up to three days. To reheat, simply set your sous vide cooker to 135-degrees F and cook the eggs for thirty minutes before serving.

Sous Vide Burgers

Cooking burger patties sous vide allows you to spend less time grilling, and more time socializing with your friends and family. Once the patties come out of the water bath, they are ready to be seared to perfection on the grill.

Ingredients:

- Ground beef, 900 g (20% fat if possible)

- Egg, one large piece (around 50 g)

- Salt

- Black pepper

Procedure:

1. If you have a meat grinder, it is highly recommended that you grind your own beef; otherwise, go for

freshly ground beef at the butcher's. Avoid frozen ground beef as much as possible, since it may no longer be fresh and give you the best results.

2. Set the water bath to 133-degrees F.

3. Put the ground beef in the bowl and add the egg; mix until egg is completely incorporated.

4. Portion beef into patties at least 200 g each. Shape patties by forming meat into a ball to remove air and then flattening it. Pinch the sides into shape using your thumbs.

5. Season beef with salt and black pepper before putting into gallon-size Ziploc bags; limit to two per bag to avoid overcrowding.

6. Cook for fifteen to thirty minutes depending on the thickness of the patty. However, it is all right if you leave them there for as long as an hour but do not exceed this time.

7. Place patties on the hot grill, sear for fifteen seconds. Flip and add cheese if desired, then cook for another thirty seconds. If cheese is added, cook an additional

fifteen seconds to melt.

Sous Vide Thin-Cut Fries

By pre-cooking the potatoes sous vide before frying them, you get fries that are crispy on the outside and fluffy and light on the inside. The secret is in the three-cooking process, in which the potatoes are cooked sous vide in brine to ensure that the outer crust is a deeper golden brown by slightly elevating its pH.

Ingredients:

- Russet potatoes, Burbank, around a half-kilogram or three unpeeled large potatoes

- Oil for cooking

Brine:

- Water, 1 kg

- Salt, 15 kg

- Glucose syrup, DE 42, 10 g (if not available, you can use 2.5 g of granulated sugar instead)

- Baking soda, 2.5 g

For seasoning:

- Kosher salt and black pepper, ground fine

Procedure:

1. Start by selecting potatoes ideal for frying. Make two bowls of brine with 1 kg water each, one with 90 kg salt and the other with 120 kg. Place potatoes in weaker brine; set aside those that float since they are too wet to fry. Place potatoes that float into the stronger brine; use those that float for your fries.

2. Peel the potatoes and submerge in water to retard browning.

3. Cut the potatoes into thin fries of around 9 mm each; return to water to prevent browning.

4. Mix ingredients to make brine.

5. Package fries in a bag with around the same weight of fries (to make them easier to handle, use 500 g of fries per bag). Make sure that the fries are in a single layer.

6. Cook the fries for around fifteen minutes until very

tender. For best results, cook until the potatoes are almost falling apart.

7. Place fries on a wire rack to cool, making sure they don't touch each other.

8. Fill a large pot around halfway with cooking oil and heat until it reaches 266-degrees F.

9. Lower the fries in small batches into the oil using a slotted spoon or strainer. Cook for around five minutes; the fries should feel firm and dry when removed from the oil.

10. Lay the cooked fries on a wire rack to dry. If not serving at once, the fries can be stored for several months in the freezer; if possible, vacuum pack them before freezing to avoid becoming rancid.

11. If you are going to serve the fries, fill a large pot with oil and heat to 374-degrees F. Make sure that the pot is big enough that the oil will not overflow when you add the fries and there is enough oil that the temperature does not fall too far when cold fries are put in.

12. Fry again until the surface turns golden brown and

the bubbles streaming from the cooking slow to a trickle, around a minute and 45 seconds.

13. Drain on paper towels to remove excess oil from fries and prevent them from being greasy.

14. Season to taste with kosher salt and black pepper. Serve. You can also serve the fries with your favorite dip.

Sous Vide Korean Pork Ribs

If you are feeling adventurous, you might want to try this delicious pork ribs recipe from South Korea. It uses sweet and spicy Hoisin sauce in the glaze to give it a distinctive taste. This recipe serves two to three.

Ingredients:

- Back Ribs, one rack

Marinade:

- Soy Sauce, 120 ml (half-cup)

- Hoisin Sauce, 80 ml (1/3-cup)

- Brown sugar, 50 g (1/4-cup)

- Sesame oil, 30 ml (two tablespoons)

- Peeled and minced garlic cloves, 4 pieces

- Peeled and grated fresh ginger, half-inch piece

- Sriracha sauce, 15 ml to 30 ml, one to two tablespoons

Garnish

- Toasted sesame seeds, 30 g (three tablespoons)

- Sliced and trimmed green onions, six bulbs

Procedure:

1. Peel off the thin membrane from the back of the ribs. Cut into individual portions.

2. Whisk all the marinade ingredients together in a bowl.

3. Place ribs in a Ziploc bag or bowl and add marinade. Toss ribs until they are completely coated in marinade. Refrigerate for around 2 – 3 hours. At around the hour – 90 minute mark, turn ribs over to ensure to ensure both sides are equally coated. Set aside

around a half-cup of the marinade.

4. Preheat water to 160-degrees F.

5. Transfer ribs to cooking pouches, around five at a time or just enough per bag that they are only one layer deep. Vacuum seal the bags.

6. Place bags in the water and let cook for eighteen hours.

7. About a half-hour before the ribs are done, make the glaze by cooking the remaining marinade in a saucepan and heating at medium/low heat; reduce heat by half to finish glaze.

8. Before ribs are done, preheat oven to 425-degrees F.

9. Remove pouches from the water and move ribs to a broiling pan using tongs.

10. Brush the ribs with glaze and cook in the oven for five minutes; repeat once more.

11. Serve with a garnish of green onions and sesame seeds.

Sous Vide Glazed Carrots

Carrot lovers will go crazy for this recipe, which produces tenderized carrots with an intense natural flavor that is enhanced by a sweet delicious glaze. This recipe produces four to six servings.

Ingredients

- Whole baby carrots, well-scrubbed or peeled, 1 pound/Medium to large carrots, one pound, peeled and cut into one-inch pieces

- Unsalted butter, 30g (two tablespoons)

- Granulated sugar, 12g (one tablespoon)

- Kosher salt

- Black pepper, freshly ground

- Chopped parsley, 15ml (one tablespoon) (optional)

Procedure

1. Preheat cooker to 183-degrees F.

2. Place ingredients and half-teaspoon of kosher salt in

a vacuum bag and seal.

3. Cook for around an hour or until carrots are fully tender.

4. Empty bag into a heavy bottomed 12-inch skillet. Cook mixture over high heat for around two minutes, stirring constantly until the liquid has turned to a shiny glaze.

5. Season with salt and pepper; add parsley if desired and serve immediately.

6. If the glaze breaks and becomes greasy, re-form glaze by adding a teaspoon of water at a time and then shaking the pan.

7. If you are not planning to cook carrots at once, they can be stored for up to a week in the refrigerator.

Sous Vide Smoky Pulled Pork Shoulder

This recipe will allow you to cook pork so tender you can literally pull it apart with your fingers. The main disadvantage is that it will take a long lead-time to cook, but the results will be more than worth the wait.

Ingredients:

- Pork butt (shoulder), bone-in or boneless, one piece of around five to seven pounds (2.25 kg to 3.25 kg)

- Kosher salt

- Liquid smoke, 3ml (half-teaspoon)

Spice Rub:

- Paprika, 50g (One-fourth cup)

- Dark brown sugar, 50g (one-fourth cup)

- Kosher salt, 35g (three tablespoons)

- Whole yellow mustard seed, 12g (one tablespoon)

- Freshly-ground black pepper, 4g (one teaspoon)

- Granulated garlic powder, 20g (two tablespoons)

- Dried oregano, 8g (one tablespoon)

- Whole coriander seed, 12g (one tablespoon)

- Red pepper flakes, 4g (one teaspoon)

Procedure:

1. Combine spice rub ingredients in a spice grinder in batches; grind to a fine powder.

2. Divide spice rub mixture in half; set aside one of the halves. Rub the mixture into the pork, pressing it firmly until it sticks.

3. Place pork in bag; add liquid smoke if desired; seal.

4. Set cooker at the desired temperature based on the level of doneness desired: if tender but sliceable, 145-degrees F, if traditional texture pulled pork, 165-degrees F.

5. Place bag in a water bath and cook for eighteen to twenty-four hours.

6. If finishing in the oven, set the temperature to 300-degrees F and place rack in middle position. Blot pork dry with paper towels then rub remaining spice mixture on the surface. Prepare wire rack by setting in a rimmed baking sheet; place pork on it and then put into the oven. Roast for around ninety minutes or until a dark, deep bark has formed.

7. If finishing on a grill, start by lighting half a chimney

with charcoal; pour out when all the coals have been lit and are covered with grey ash. Arrange coal on one side of the grill, and then place grate in place then cover grill; preheat for five minutes. Prepare pork as described in step 6 and then place pork on the grill's cooler side. Add four to five chunks of hardwood to the hotter side of grill; cover grill and let pork smoke. Make sure the temperature is maintained at a range of 275-degrees F to 300-degrees F by adjusting vents; while cooking add 2 to 3 chunks twice. Smoke for around 90 minutes or until a bark has formed.

8. Transfer pork to bowl or cutting board. Depending on the level of doneness, shred pork with two forks or slice with a knife into bite-sized pieces. Serve immediately with your favorite barbecue sauce.

9. If pork will not be cooked at once, it can be kept in the refrigerator for as long as a week after sous vide.

Sous Vide Spanish-Style Paprika Shrimp

There are a number of advantages to cooking shrimp sous vide including being able to infuse them with flavor while they are cooking and getting textures that you wouldn't be able to get with traditional cooking methods.

This recipe gives you shrimp infused with Mediterranean flavors including spicy paprika, garlic, and extra-virgin coconut oil. Another trick to cooking shrimp sous vide is tossing it with baking soda to give it a firmer texture.

Depending on the texture you want, there are four cooking temperatures you can choose:

- Semi-raw and translucent, with a buttery, soft texture – 125-degrees F

- Very tender and almost opaque, with a touch of firmness – 130-degrees F

- Tender, juicy and moist, and scarcely opaque - 135-degrees F

- Conventional poached texture, with juicy, crisp bite and good bounce – 140-degrees F

Ingredients:

- Large shrimp, peeled, 1 ½-pound (700 g)

- Baking soda, half-teaspoon

- Kosher salt

- Extra-virgin olive oil, 90 ml (six tablespoons)

- Garlic, six thinly sliced medium cloves

- Spanish paprika, 6 g (one tablespoon)

- Sherry, 45 ml (three tablespoons)

- Bay leaves, two pieces

- Butter, 30 g (two tablespoons)

- Sherry vinegar, 6 ml (1 ½-tablespoons)

Procedure:

1. Set sous vide cooker temperature based on the desired texture.

2. Toss shrimp in a large bowl with baking soda and half-teaspoon kosher salt; set aside.

3. Heat the garlic and olive oil over medium heat in a large skillet. Cook for around three minutes, constantly stirring, until garlic sizzles and softens but does not turn brown. Add bay leaves and paprika, cook for another thirty seconds, constantly stirring

until it becomes fragrant. Then add the sherry and sherry vinegar, and cook at high for around two minutes, until the sauce begins to emulsify and the liquid is reduced. Remove skillet from heat and stir in butter. Season with salt to taste and let cool for around five minutes.

4. Place shrimp in the vacuum bag or heavy-duty sealer bag; pour in garlic/olive oil mixture and then remove all the air using displacement method or vacuum sealer. Press bag so shrimp are arranged in a single layer.

5. Place bag in a water bath and cook for at least fifteen minutes but no more than an hour.

6. Pour shrimp into a warmed bowl and serve with crusty bread for sopping up excess sauce.

Sous Vide Poached Shrimp

Here's a recipe for traditional poached shrimp with a sous vide twist: not only will you enjoy more flavorful shrimp, you can infuse it with butter while cooking to add extra flavor.

Cooking temperature chart:

- Semi-raw and translucent, with a buttery, soft texture – 125-degrees F

- Very tender and almost opaque, with a touch of firmness – 130-degrees F

- Tender, juicy and moist, and scarcely opaque - 135-degrees F

- Conventional poached texture, with juicy, crisp bite and good bounce – 140-degrees F

Ingredients:

- Large shrimp, peeled, 1 ½-pound (700 g)

- Baking soda, half-teaspoon

- Kosher salt

- Extra-virgin olive oil or butter (optional)

- Aromatics such as garlic, parsley or shallots (optional)

Procedure:

1. Use temperature chart to choose the cooking temperature. Set water bath to the desired temperature.

2. In a large bowl, toss shrimp with kosher salt and baking soda. Place in a heavy-duty Ziploc bag or vacuum bag; if desired add butter or olive oil and aromatics.

3. Cook for a minimum of fifteen minutes to no more than an hour.

4. Serve at once or chill first then serve cold.

Sous Vide Steaks

Cooking steaks sous vide gives you perfectly even results through slow cooking that you can replicate every time. After cooking, you can finish the steaks on a grill or pan to give it a dark crust.

Temperature Cooking Chart:

Butcher's Cut/Tenderloin/T-Bone/Porterhouse/Strip

- Very Rare to Rare – 120-degrees F to 128-degrees F – one hour to 2 ½-hours

- Medium Rare – 129-degrees F to 134-degrees F – one

hour to four hours (or no more than 2 ½-hours if cooked at less than 130-degrees F)

- Medium – 135-degrees F to 144-degrees F - one to four hours

- Medium-well – 145-degrees F to 155-degrees F – one hour to 3 ½-hours

- Well Done – 156-degrees F and up – one hour to three hours

Tenderloin

- Very Rare to Rare – 120-degrees F to 128-degrees F – 45 minutes to 2 ½-hours

- Medium Rare – 129-degrees F to 134-degrees F – 45 minutes to four hours (or no more than 2 ½-hours if cooked at less than 130-degrees F)

- Medium – 135-degrees F to 144-degrees F – 45 minutes to four hours

- Medium-well – 145-degrees F to 155-degrees F – 45 minutes to 3 ½-hours

- Well Done – 156-degrees F and up – one hour to

three hours

Ingredients:

- Steaks, two (1 ½-inch to 2 inch thick) pieces (porter-house, T-bone, strip or ribeye) or four (6 to 8 oz.) pieces tenderloin

- Freshly ground black pepper and kosher salt

- Canola oil, two tablespoons

- Butter, two tablespoons

- Rosemary or thyme, two sprigs (optional)

- Garlic, two cloves (optional)

- Shallots, two pieces, thinly sliced (optional)

Procedure:

1. Preheat sous vide cooker to the desired temperature. Season steaks with salt and pepper and place in bag with spices if desired. Seal bags then place in water bath for appropriate cooking time. Pat dry thoroughly before cooking.

2. If using a pan to finish, open your windows first since

cooking will produce smoke. Place canola, rice bran or vegetable oil in a stainless steel or cast iron skillet and put on the hottest burner; preheat until oil starts to smoke. Put the steak in the skillet (if desired, add one tablespoon butter or omit to get a cleaner-tasting sear), and then cook one side for fifteen to thirty seconds and then flip and cook for fifteen to thirty seconds. Keep flipping the steak for around ninety seconds until the desired sear is achieved. If you did not add butter earlier, you can do so thirty seconds before steak is done. Serve immediately.

3. If you are using a charcoal grill, take a chimney full of charcoal and light it; when all the charcoal is covered in a light grey ash arrange the coals on one side of the grate. If using gas-fired grill then set half the burners to the highest setting, and then cover and preheat for ten minutes.

4. Place cooking grate, cover grill and preheat for five minutes. Clean and oil the grate then place steak on the hot side. Cook steak for around ninety seconds, turning it over every fifteen to thirty seconds until rich, deep crust has formed. If the fire flares up due

to dripping fat, transfer steak to cooler side or suffoc-
ate fire by closing lid until it dies out.

5. Transfer steak to serving platter or cutting board and
   serve immediately.

Sous Vide Yoghurt

The main advantage of using sous vide to make yogurt is
that you can greatly shorten the process from several days
to just a few hours. It yields around five servings. However,
you will need cooking jars rather than sealable bags.

Ingredients:

- Whole milk, 800 g

- Live culture yogurt, 40 g

Procedure:

1. Preheat sous vide cooker to 109-degrees F.

2. In a pot warm milk to 180-degrees F over low heat.
   While heating, run a spatula around the bottom to
   ensure the milk doesn't scald. Remove from heat and
   cool down; alternatively, you can prepare an ice bath

to cool down the milk more quickly. The final temperature of the milk should be 110-degrees F.

3. Place live culture yogurt in a bowl with a spoon. Add some of the milk and then stir until smooth. Add the remaining milk and then stir mixture until fully combined.

4. Pour mixture into a one-liter jar or several smaller jars. Screw lids on tightly.

5. Transfer jars to the water bath. Let stay for at least five hours.

6. Remove jars from water and transfer to refrigerator. Let sit overnight before eating.

Sous Vide Crème Brule

One of the biggest challenges in preparing Crème Brule using traditional methods is that there is a risk it will curdle if the internal temperature goes above 185-degrees F. Sous vide avoids this problem by cooking the custards at a precise temperature.

To add that delicious final touch, a blowtorch is used to create a layer of golden-brown caramelized sugar before serving. You will need canning jars instead of sealable packages for this recipe.

Ingredients:

- Egg yolks, eleven or around 160 g

- Granulated sugar, 90 g

- Heavy cream, 600 g

- Salt, 3 g

Procedure:

1. Preheat sous vide cooker to 176-degrees F.

2. In a bowl, combine egg yolks, salt, and sugar; whisk mixture until smooth.

3. If desired, heat cream in a pot to 158-degrees F (optional); otherwise, pour cream into egg yolk mixture. Introduce the cream slowly to avoid curdling, then gradually increase pour rate.

4. Strain mixture using a fine mesh strainer. Let rest for around a half-hour to allow bubbles to dissipate. Any remaining bubbles on the surface can be skimmed

away.

5. Place some 150 g of custard mixture per jar; avoid pouring too quickly or from too high a level so bubbles won't form on the surface.

6. Just barely close the lids in such a way that you can still open them with your fingertips. This is important since it allows air to escape from the jars. If the lid is closed too tight, the air pressure inside the jar may cause it to crack.

7. Place jars in water bath and cook for an hour.

8. Remove from water and let rest at room temperature.

9. Prepare an ice bath, then transfer the jars to it and chill. Once the jars are cold, tighten the lids and transfer to refrigerator. The Crème Brule will last for around a week.

To create caramelized top layer:

1. Open the jar; if condensation has formed on top of the custard, remove by dabbing with the corner of a paper towel.

2. Dust a layer of granulated sugar on top using your fingers or a small sieve; the more sugar, the more crunchy and caramelized the layer will be.

3. Turn the blowtorch on at low-gas release. Hold the torch in your dominant hand and the jar in the other; aim the flame at the custard while rotating the jar with your hand. Move the torch closer and farther to control the heat; the distance between the torch and the jar should range from 10 inches to 24 inches.

4. When the layer has turned the desired color, let the sugar set for five minutes before eating to allow it to achieve maximum crunchiness.

Sous Vide Lemon Curd

This recipe cooks the ingredients sous vide to create an oozy, soft curd.

Ingredients:

- Lemons, four pieces

- Butter, 200 g

- Sugar, 175 g (dextrose can also be used)

- Egg yolks, eight pieces or around 120 g

- Citric acid, 5 g

- Salt, 1 g

- 180-bloom gelatin, 13 g (optional)

- Ice water

Procedure:

1. Preheat water to 167-degrees F.

2. Use lemons to create 10 g of zest and 150 g of lemon juice (if you don't know how to make zest, see instructions below).

3. Combine ingredients along with lemon zest in a small Ziploc bag or sous vide pouch. If you would like it to be less sweet, you can replace it with dextrose. You can also add gelatin if you want the curd to have a texture that is more jam-like.

4. Cook for one hour.

5. Transfer curd to a blender and blend on high for thirty to sixty seconds, until the mixture is fully emul-

sified. You should stop blending when the curd stops changing color, since as you blend the color will lighten.

6. If there are air bubbles, you can remove them by transferring the curd to chamber sealer or knock the bowl on the counter several times.

7. To chill, transfer the curd to bowl and place in ice bath.

To make lemon zest:

1. With a paring knife, cut strips of zest from the skin of the lemon but make sure that you avoid too much pith; leaving too much pit can cause the zest to taste bitter. You can do this by cutting the top and bottom of the lemon so you can see where the pith is.

2. Place the knife on the edge of the skin. Guide the knife down following the curve of the skin. Chop it finely to use in the recipe above or you can leave it in strips for other uses.

3. If you have a grater, you can create zest by lightly grazing the skin, either moving in a circular motion

or in strips.

Sous Vide Crispy Chicken with Cheddar Broccoli Sauce

This delicious dish will surely be a staple in your household once you've tried it.

Ingredients:

- Chicken legs, 4 pieces, skin-on

- Broccoli Cheddar Sauce:

- Broccoli, one whole head

- Sweet onion, half piece, medium diced

- Unsalted butter, 40 g

- Salt, 5 g

- Minced garlic, 4 g

- White wine, 82 g

- Heavy cream, 340 g

- Aged white cheddar, 100 g

- Black pepper to taste

- White button mushrooms, six pieces cut into quarters (optional)

Procedure:

To make the sauce:

1. Trim off broccoli florets with a paring knife; set aside. Chop remainder roughly.

2. Combine chopped broccoli stems and leavings with onion in food processor and pulse until mixture is finely minced.

3. Place butter, garlic, and salt along with onion-broccoli mixture in a pot and cook slowly over medium-high heat. Let sweat until garlic and onions have cooked down and are fragrant, around six minutes.

4. Add white wine and reduce; when almost no clear liquid is left, add cheese and cream. Reduce until it has achieved a fondue-like consistency; avoid scorching by whisking frequently (for this recipe, however, it should only be reduced halfway). Let sit until you are ready to serve.

5. Heat sauce and reduce until it has reached a thick consistency.

6. Add the broccoli florets and mushrooms (optional); reduce heat to low. Cover.

7. Season with black pepper

To make chicken:

1. Heat water to 158-degrees F.

2. Place chicken legs in Ziploc bag with some oil.

3. Immerse in water and cook for around an hour.

4. Thoroughly pat dry using paper towels.

5. Generously add enough oil to a cast-iron skillet or non-stick pan to ensure it is covered. Heat until the oil starts to smoke and then put thighs in a pan with skin side down using tongs.

6. Sear for around a minute, until skin is golden brown. Season with salt to taste.

7. To serve, place a mound of the sauce onto plate or bowl, and lightly drizzle with extra-virgin olive oil.

8. Place a thigh on top of sauce; if desired, garnish with flat leaf parsley.

9. If desired, you can serve on preheated dishes. Simply place the serving dishes in an oven that has been set to lowest setting; remove when ready to serve.

10 - Conclusion

Thank you for buying this book!

I hope that this book was useful in helping you learn to cook sous vide. Although this cooking technique may seem odd at first, once you've gotten used to preparing food this way, you'll realize how easy it actually is and how much better food made this way tastes.

Thank you again and good luck!

Book 2 - Sous Vide

Delicious Recipes For Easy Cooking At Home (Cooking Through Science, Recipe Book, Modern Meals, Ultimate Guide)

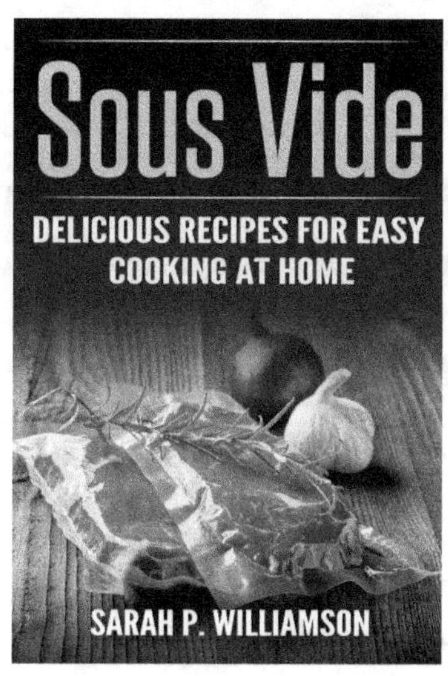

1 - Introduction

What is sous vide?

Basically, sous vide is a French method of cooking wherein the ingredients are placed in a food-grade plastic bag and vacuum sealed. Then, it is placed in a water bath heated at precisely the right temperature and slow cooked to perfection. That might sound a bit complicated at first, but in reality, it is simpler and easier than stove-top or oven cooking.

How is it better than the other cooking methods?

Well, it ensures that the food is properly cooked – you no longer have to worry about over- or under-cooking at all! Best of all, you do not even have to wait hand and foot on your food as it cooks; all you need is a timer to remind you when to take it out.

At this point, you might be wondering why sous vide is not as popular when it is more effective. The answer is that some people think only chefs from Michelin star restaurants are skilled at sous vide cooking. However, this book is here to prove you wrong.

Anyone – whether you are indeed a skilled chef or a dedicated homemaker – can do sous vide. All you need in your kitchen are two pieces of equipment and this cookbook to help you get started.

In this book, you will learn how sous vide works, what its benefits are, how to be familiar with your sous vide equipment, and the basic sous vide cooking guidelines. Most important of all is the collection of sous vide recipes for vegetables, poultry, seafood, red meat, and desserts that you can try out in your kitchen.

Sous vide is all about cooking food at the precise temperature. As a result, you will get the optimal flavor, texture, and nutritional value of your food. So go ahead, delve into the world of sous vide, and turn to the first chapter now!

How Sous Vide Works

There is only one main element that sets the difference between cooked foods and the raw ingredient, and that is heat. Heat transforms a dry and dull piece of carrot into something crisp, tender and mealy. It alters a doughy mixture of flour, sugar, eggs, butter, and salt into a fluffy and sweet cake.

However, to obtain the best results one must not just submit the ingredients to heat at any level but rather to precision heating. Otherwise, the chemicals in the ingredients when exposed to too much or too little heat would result in flavors and textures that are not as desirable.

The art of carefully manipulating the heat to prepare the food is necessary for sous vide, the modern form of the medieval French water bath food preparation system called bain-marie. 'Sous vide' literally translates to "under vacuum," and was discovered in 1972 by French biochemist and microbiologist Bruno Goussault.

When Goussault was tasked by a European fast-food chain called Wimpy's to find a cheap way to make tough beef cuts tender and juicy, what he did was vacuum-pack the meat in a plastic bag and then give it a water bath in the oven set to 60 °C (or 140 °F).

Around the 1980s, the cooking method penetrated the United States but did not catch on immediately because it was expensive, unusual, and was thought to have safety issues as questioned by the Food and Drug Administration. It was not until French chef Gérard Bertholon described it in detail to the top American chefs in 2000 when it was recognized as a safe, effective, and efficient way to cooking.

To apply sous vide, you will need to use two special pieces of equipment. The first one is a vacuum-packing appliance that allows you to tightly seal the food inside a plastic bag. This eliminates any air pockets inside the plastic bag and ensures that the food is compressed. Therefore, once it is immersed in the water the food will be heated evenly without it being in direct contact with the water.

The second device is referred to as the immersion circulator, and it is used to heat the food at the ideal temperature. It has the functions of a thermometer, pump, and heater to heat the food at precisely the right level and to keep the water circulating around the food to ensure even heating.

At this point, you may be wondering how much heat is required in sous vide. To answer your query, sous vide cooking usually makes use of heat that is just enough to precisely cook the food and no more than that. To be specific, the water in sous vide rarely goes beyond 85 °C (or 185 °F), a temperature that is below simmering point.

Therefore, it is different than the kind of heat food is exposed to when placed inside an oven or a pan of hot oil, because in the latter two, the outer portion of the food would be overcooked by the time the heat reaches the food's core.

With sous vide, the result is food that is perfectly cooked. A single degree in Celsius or two to three degrees in Fahrenheit make a huge impact on the over- or under-doneness of the food. For instance, an egg that is boiled at 60 °C (or 140 °F) would result in a gooey consistency, but when it is cooked at 62.8 °C (or 145 °F) the result is a firm yolk with a relatively tender white.

The idea of setting the exact temperature to heat the food in precisely the right way might sound complicated, but in truth, it makes life so much easier. For example, let us say you want to cook your meat to an internal temperature of exactly 60 °C (or 140 °F), all you have to do is set the immersion circulator to heat it at exactly to that level of temperature.

After around 30 minutes, the result would be perfectly cooked medium rare meat that will retain the same temperature until it is served. Of course, the same cannot be applied if you are to sauté, grill, braise, or even bake it.

As you can see, sous vide is anything but unusual and strange; it is a cooking method that guarantees precision. It is for those who only want to enjoy the best food in every meal, prepared in a simple and straightforward way, and cooked to perfection.

2 - Choosing Your Sous Vide Equipment

Whether you are the head chef of a five-star restaurant or a homemaker who prides him or herself on providing only the best quality meals for the family, you can add the two pieces of equipment needed for sous vide.

As soon as you are ready to make the investment, you are going to be looking for a chamber vacuum-packing machine and an immersion circulator. This chapter will discuss with you in detail the purpose of the two and how you can find one of each for your needs.

The Chamber Vacuum-Packing Machine

The purpose of the chamber vacuum-packing machine or the vacuum packer is to suck the air out of the food-grade plastic bag that contains your food and then seals it. By removing the air, the food will be heated at the precise level you want it and at the same time, the food will not be as susceptible to freezer burn or spoilage thus enhancing its shelf life.

Those who wish to do sous vide at home for oneself or the family will do well with the countertop model which stands at approximately 12 inches high with a width of 18 inches and a depth of 12 inches.

For those who need an industrial type of model, this equipment comes in stand-alone versions with their own set of wheels for easy maneuvering in a five-star kitchen. Typically, the chamber vacuum-packing machine has a lid that is transparent shaped like a dome to enable you to see what is going on inside as it heats the food.

To use this piece of equipment, all you need to do is place the food inside the plastic bag and then put it inside its chamber. Then, as soon as you turn on the machine it will suck the air out of the bag and seal it. Naturally, the amount of pressure can be controlled because vacuum-sealing delicate pieces such as fish and poultry require lower pressure than sealing tough meats and hard root vegetables.

The great thing about this machine is it can also seal liquid ingredients, including marinades, oils, and stock. However, not all models are built in the same way so you should take into consideration the machine's ability to seal liquids before making your purchase.

Now, when it comes to choosing the right plastic bags, you

should find ones that are at least 0.003 inches thick, or durable enough so as not to become damaged during the sealing process. You must also make sure to choose bags that are made with food-grade plastic in that they are safe when exposed to 100 °C (or 212 °F), or at boiling temperature.

The Immersion Circulator

All models of this type of equipment include three fundamental parts: a heating tool that increases the temperature of the water, a temperature moderator that sets the heating tool to maintain the precise temperature you set it, and a pump that causes the water to circulate inside the machine.

To use an immersion circulator, all you need to do is attach it to your cooking vessel, plug it in, and turn it on. After that, you set it to the temperature you want the food to be cooked in and let it do its job.

Now, no one should confuse the use of the immersion circulator as an alternative to other cooking methods. Rather, it should be treated as a complementary step in preparing the food. For example, after you have heated your short ribs at exactly 57.2 °C (or 135 °F) for 48 hours using the immersion circulator, you can then sear them on a hot pan to get that perfectly crisp coating before serving.

3 - Sous Vide Basic Cooking Guidelines

Before you start sous vide cooking, there are specific guidelines to keep in mind. The first set of guidelines has to do with the roles of your two pieces of sous vide equipment. The second set is made up of the four fundamental sous vide methods you can apply to your food. The third and highly important set involves the safety guidelines to religiously abide by when doing sous vide cooking.

This chapter will discuss both guidelines so that you can then transition to the recipes with ease and confidence.

The Three Factors: Pressure, Temperature and Time

Three factors affect the results of your sous vide cooking, and these are pressure, temperature, and time. It is important to understand the role of each so that you will get the results you want, which is why this chapter is dedicated to them.

Pressure: seal the food properly

The pressure applied by your chamber vacuum-packing machine has an impact on the results of your sous vide. It should be the perfect balance between an even compression (to eliminate air pockets) and controlled pressure (to avoid crushing any delicate parts of the food or puncturing the bag).

The standard chamber vacuum-packing machine has two gauges: the first one is to measure out the amount of pressure and the second one is to control the length of time of packing.

Therefore, while the recipes in this book call for general settings (low, medium and high) when applying pressure, you must first read the manufacturer's manual for your particular model so that you can adjust your settings accordingly.

Now, as for the length of time to which you set the machine in applying pressure to your bag, you must take into consideration the thickness and overall quality of the plastic bag you are using. The general rule is that thicker bags require more heat.

The hardness of the food also affects your decision in applying pressure to it. For example, root vegetables such as potatoes and carrots need high pressure to ensure that the bag is completely hugging them and ensuring an even heat distribution once they undergo heating. On the other hand, delicate foods such as white fish require a lot less pressure so that they do not become crushed and unpalatable.

It is important to remember that the food should always be chilled when you are packing and sealing it. Many chefs forget this make this mistake and the results obviously are from perfect. The reason why food must always be cold is that water vaporizes when submitted to low-pressure situations. Thus, if warm food is placed inside the machine, the food will become dry and less desirable.

If you plan to cook sous vide something that has been seared beforehand, you should, therefore, chill it afterward (ideally for 8 hours, or overnight) before you seal it. To be specific, the food should be below 6 °C (or 42.8 °F).

Temperature: sous vide heat precision

Sous vide requires a temperature level of no more than 85 °C (or 185 °F), which is below simmering water. Hard vegetables are usually submerged at this level to tenderize them.

Meats are typically exposed to temperature levels between 60 and 70 °C (or 140 and 160 °F) depending on their thickness, consistency, and the results you want to achieve. Fish, on the other hand, are more delicate and therefore are submerged at a temperature that is roughly 6.6 °C (or 11.9 °F) lower than most meats. Delicate fish such as dory, for example, are cooked at 60 °C (or 140 °F).

Tender meats such as chicken breasts are usually submerged at 62 °C temperature (or 143.6 °F), while thighs are at 64 °C (or 147.2 °F). Of course, these are not set in stone, but rather should be regarded as general guidelines. For instance, seared chicken breasts may require shorter sous vide cooking time than their raw counterpart.

Time: How long it takes

The biggest difference between sous vide and other cooking methods is in how it maintains the temperature of the food as it cooks. In a traditional cooking method, such as boiling, the food needs to be monitored and timed carefully. Otherwise, the food will come out undercooked and tough or overcooked and soggy.

Sous vide cooking, on the other hand, will maintain the desired internal temperature of the food as soon as it reaches it. Therefore, you can remove it from the water at any time and to your convenience. However, it does not mean there is no limit to the length of time it stays in the water, for if it is overexposed it will affect the texture of the food.

4 - The Four Fundamental Sous Vide Methods

Sous vide is applied to achieve at least one of its four purposes, namely Storage, Marination, Cooking, and Compression. Being able to apply all four will ensure that you are maximizing the equipment you have invested on and also guarantee the maintenance of the food in its highest quality form.

Storage

Simply put, food that is vacuum sealed will have a significantly longer shelf life, especially in the refrigerator or freezer, compared to food that is loosely packed or even stored in airtight containers. The sous vide technique eliminates the oxygen within the environment of the food, thus inhibiting the development of bacteria that can spoil it.

Aside from extending the food's shelf life, sous vide food will not become discolored because oxidation will not transpire. This is especially important in sliced fruits and vegetables because if exposed parts come into contact with the oxygen they will quickly lose their color, flavor, and nutritional value.

It is also worth noting that vacuum sealed foods stored in the freezer will also be able to retain natural moisture because it cannot escape from its tight environment. As a result, freezer burn can be prevented.

Marination

All good cooks would agree that marinating is an essential cooking process. It adds more depth, texture, and flavor to the food and it opens you up to a wide variety of food possibilities.

Now, placing your food and the marinade in the plastic bag and then applying sous vide will make the distribution of the marinade more even. Therefore, it will strengthen the potency of your marinade.

Vacuum sealed marinated food is also easier to manage and store in the refrigerator compared to marinating in bulky containers. Thus, you will not only be able to marinate more ingredients but also organize them efficiently.

Cooking

The primary sous vide technique is cooking, without a doubt, and there are three main strategies to apply it: à la minute or short time cooking, long time cooking (which can last for a number of days), and fruit and vegetable cooking.

Delicate food such as fish usually calls for short time cooking, which can be as short as 10 minutes, and then is served right afterwards. Tough meats such as beef and pork require longer cooking time to ensure tenderness. Vegetables generally require between half an hour to 1 hour and 30 minutes cooking time.

Compression

Mark Hopper, the chef de cuisine at Bouchon in Las Vegas, discovered the fourth and latest sous vide strategy of Compression. This particular strategy is applied to alter the food's texture, especially with porous fruit such as melons. Compression calls for the use of high pressure to change the lightness of the fruit into one that is denser and more "compact."

Aside from changing the texture of the food, compression also enables the cook to change its shape and to keep it that way. This process is known as "setting" and it helps you store food in the shape you desire. For example, pork loin wrapped in bacon through sous vide compression can easily maintain its shapeliness and stored accordingly before it is cooked using another method.

5 - Sous Vide Safety Guidelines

At this point, you must be quite excited to venture the world of sous vide, but before you do so, you must master the basic guidelines of food safety for obvious reasons. This part shows you the rules you must keep in mind whenever you wish to apply sous vide.

The first rule has to do with preventing the development of harmful pathogens in your food, namely E. coli, salmonella, Clostridium botulinum, and so on. These types of bacteria, unfortunately, thrive in anaerobic (zero oxygen) environments which can make the vacuum-sealed back their perfect ecosystem.

If the bag is contaminated and exposed to warm water (or a temperature between 40 and 50 °C or 100 and 120 °F), they will multiply to potentially fatal levels.

To keep these harmful pathogens from proliferating in your vacuum sealed bags, you should always keep the food cold and prevent it from staying in that temperature or in room temperature for too long. You should also make sure to vacuum seal fresh foods, especially meats, and to cook them soon after you have bought them.

It is also important to note that you should not expose food sealed sous vide to a temperature between 4.4 and 60 °C (or 40 and 140 °F) for over 4 hours. Therefore, as soon as the chilled food is vacuum-sealed, you should proceed to cook or store it right away.

The food you want to sous vide has been heated or seared, you can place it in a bowl and then give the bowl an ice bath to quickly cool down the temperature of the food. To prepare an ice bath, simply fill a large basin halfway with water and the remaining half with ice, and then place the container of hot food on top to chill it quickly.

Once sufficiently chilled, you can then vacuum seal it and store it at 3.3 °C (or 38 °F) or lower. Also, do note that foods you plan to cook for over 3 days should be stored in the freezer instead of the refrigerator.

Now, with all these guidelines in mind, you can confidently proceed to make full use of your sous vide equipment and prepare your meals in precisely the way you want them to be.

6 - Fruit and Vegetable Recipes

Pickled Beets

Total Preparation Time: 2 hours

Temperature: 85 °C (or 185 °F)

Number of Servings: 6

You will need:

- 450 grans beets, sliced into ½ inch pieces

- 1 garlic clove, peeled and diced

- ¾ Serrano pepper, seeded

- 1 cup white wine vinegar

- 1 cup filtered water

- 3 Tbsp. pickling salt

How to prepare:

1. Combine the white wine vinegar, filtered water, and pickling salt in a saucepan and place over a high flame. Bring to a boil, then reduce to simmer. Continue to simmer, stirring frequently, until the salt is

dissolved.

2. Turn off the heat and set aside to cool.

3. Combine the beets, Serrano pepper, and garlic into a food-grade plastic bag. Strain the brine and pour into the bag, then vacuum seal to medium. Place in the refrigerator and chill until ready to cook.

4. Set the sous vide immersion circulator to the desired temperature level.'

5. Once the sous vide water has reached the desired temperature level, add the vacuum sealed bag of beets and cook for 40 minutes.

6. After cooking, transfer the beets to an ice bath to cool to room temperature. Serve right away or store in the refrigerator for up to 12 months.

Artichokes In Herbed Vinaigrette

Total Preparation Time: 1 hour and 30 minutes

Temperature: 85 °C (or 185 °F)

Number of Servings:

You will need:

- 3 globe artichoke hearts

- 12 violet artichokes, trimmed

- 3 garlic cloves, crushed, unpeeled

- 3 fresh thyme sprigs

- 3 fresh rosemary sprigs

- 3 bay leaves

- 12 black peppercorns

- 300 grams extra virgin olive oil

- 100 grams champagne vinegar

- 6 grams sea salt

How to prepare:

Arrange the globe artichokes in a single layer in a large plastic bag and the violet artichokes in another bag. Make sure they do not overlap to ensure an even distribution.

Divide the garlic cloves, rosemary, thyme, bay leaves, and peppercorns between two tea bags and seal. Place one bag into each plastic bag.

Meanwhile, combine the olive oil, salt, and champagne vinegar very well then divide the two between the two bags. Vacuum seal the bags set to medium.

Cook the smaller artichokes in the desired temperature for about 45 minutes, and the larger artichokes for about 1 hour and 15 minutes, or until tender.

Once the artichokes are tender, place the bags of artichokes in an ice bath until completely chilled. Serve right away or refrigerate for up to 3 days.

Caramelized Herbed Fennel

Total Preparation Time: 1 hour

Temperature: 85 °C (or 185 °F)

Number of Servings: 4 to 6

You will need:

- 3 medium fennel bulbs

- 12 small or baby fennel bulbs

- 150 grams extra virgin olive oil

- 75 grams Pernod

- 5 grams caraway seeds

- 3 fresh thyme sprigs

- 3 fresh tarragon sprigs

- 3 bay leaves

- 3 star anise

- Sea salt, as needed

- Olive oil, as needed

How to prepare:

1. Start by trimming off the root ends of the fennel bulbs. Slice the tops off and save the fronds. Then, discard the outermost layers of the medium fennel bulbs. Slice the medium fennel bulbs into half-inch wedges then set aside.

2. Slice off the dark ends of the baby or small fennel bulbs on the diagonal. Then, make an incision in the bottom of each baby or small fennel bulb.

3. Divide the thyme, tarragon, star anise, bay leaves, and caraway seeds between two tea bags and place one bag into two separate plastic bags. Place the medium fennel bulb wedges in one bag and the small or baby fennel bulbs in the other. Then, vacuum seal both bags set to medium.

4. Cook the fennel bulbs at the desired temperature for about 45 minutes or until the fennel bulbs are tender. Then, chill both bags of fennel bulbs using an ice bath.

5. Once the fennel bulbs are ready, place a wok or skillet over medium flame and add enough olive oil to coat. Add the fennel wedges and sauté until caramelized. Then, place on a plate lined with paper towels to drain.

6. Finely chop the fennel fronds and set aside. Then, arrange the fennel bulbs on a platter and season to taste with salt. Top the fennel bulbs with the chopped fronds and serve right away.

Glazed Cipollini And Pearl Onion Salad

Total Preparation Time: 1 hour

6 - FRUIT AND VEGETABLE RECIPES

Temperature: 61 °C (or 142 °F)

Number of Servings:

You will need:

- 16 white pearl onions, peeled

- 12 red pearl onions, peeled

- 12 cipollini, peeled

- 100 grams cold water

- 45 grams cold unsalted water

- 25 grams champagne vinegar

- 25 grams red wine vinegar

- 25 grams canola oil

- 9 grams granulated sugar

- 9 grams sea salt

- Fleur de sel, to taste

- Chopped fresh chives, to garnish

How to prepare:

1. To prepare the pearl onions, trim them but leave enough to keep them bunched together. Slice the tops of the cipollini onions.

2. Prepare three plastic bags and add cipollini in the first, red pearl onions in the second, and white pearl onions in the third. Divide the water, salt, and sugar among the three bags, then add the oil to the bag of cipollini. Divide the butter between the two bags of pearl onions. Vacuum pack all three bags set to medium.

3. Once vacuum sealed, cook all three at the desired temperature level for 40 minutes, or until tender. Then, chill using an ice bath.

4. After the onions are chilled, drain the cipollini and blot dry with paper towels. Meanwhile, place the white and red pearl onions into separate saucepans along with their liquids. Simmer until the liquids are reduced slightly then pour in the champagne vinegar over the white pearl onions and the red wine vinegar over the red pearl onions. Simmer until the liquids become syrupy, stirring to coat the red onions over them.

5. To serve, arrange the cipollini and red and white pearl onions on a plate. Season to taste with fleur de sel, top with chives and serve right away.

Sous Vide Rhubarb And Asparagus

Total Preparation Time: 1 hour

Temperature: 61°C (or 141.8 °F) for the rhubarb and 85 °C (or 185 °F) for the asparagus

Number of Servings: 6

You will need:

For the rhubarb:

- 6 stalks rhubarb

- 3 strips freshly peeled orange zest

- 45 grams cold freshly squeezed orange juice

- 45 grams red wine vinegar

- 45 grams granulated sugar

For the asparagus:

- 12 large asparagus spears (white or green)

- 55 grams cold milk

- Granulated sugar, as needed

- Sea salt, as needed

- Extra virgin olive oil, as needed

- Champagne vinegar, as needed

- Fleur de sel, as needed

How to prepare:

1. Snap off the tough ends of the asparagus spears then peel them and trim the ends to ensure all the spears are of equal length.

2. Place the spears in a plastic bag in a single layer with the tips facing upward. Sprinkle in some granulated sugar and then pour in the milk. Vacuum seal set to medium-high.

3. Cook the asparagus spears at the desired temperature level for 30 minutes or until tender. Then transfer to an ice bath.

4. Meanwhile, blot the rhubarb thoroughly with damp paper towels. Then, trim the stalks until they all are the same length. Arrange all the stalks in a plastic bag in a single layer, then vacuum seal on medium high.

5. Cook the rhubarb to the desired temperature level for 20 minutes, or until they are tender. Then, take the bag out of the water and set aside to cool to room temperature.

6. Once the asparagus and rhubarb are ready, drain both. Rinse the asparagus using cold water and slice the ends off on the diagonal. Slice the spears on the diagonal into bite-sized pieces and place on a serving plate.

7. Blot the rhubarb dry and slice into ¼ inch thick and 1 ½ inch long pieces. Arrange with the asparagus on the platter.

8. Drizzle some olive oil and champagne vinegar over the rhubarb and asparagus then top with fleur de sel. Serve right away.

Sweet And Wild Spring Onion Salad With Special Sour Cream Sauce

Total Preparation Time: 6 hours AND 30 minutes

Temperature: 85 °C (or 185 °F)

Number of Servings: 6

You will need:

For the sweet onion:

- 2 large sweet onions, sliced thinly (about 1/6 inch)

- 35 grams organic vegetable stock, chilled

- 15 grams champagne vinegar

- Extra virgin olive oil, as needed

- Sea salt, as needed

- Freshly ground white pepper, as needed

For the pickled wild spring onion:

- 75 grams granulated sugar

- 75 grams filtered water

- 75 grams champagne vinegar

- 12 wild spring onions, blanched

For the sauce:

- 450 grams white onion, thinly sliced (about 1/8 inch)

- 150 grams organic vegetable stock, chilled

- 75 grams cold heavy cream

- 75 grams canola oil

- 40 grams champagne vinegar

- Chopped fresh chives, to garnish

- Japanese mustard greens, to garnish

How to prepare:

1. First, make the sauce by mixing together all the ingredients in a plastic bag and then vacuum seal on medium high. Once sealed, cook for 6 hours using the desired temperature level, or until the onion is extra tender.

2. Transfer the mixture to a food processor and blend

until smooth. Pour into a container and refrigerate until ready to serve.

3. To prepare the sweet onion, place a grill pan over medium-high flame and heat through. Once hot, add the onion slices and heat until seared. Transfer to a container, cover, and refrigerate until chilled.

4. Once chilled, transfer the sliced sweet onion into a plastic bag and add the vegetable stock and vinegar for them. Vacuum seal set to medium. Then, cook sous vide for 30 minutes at the desired temperature. Once cooked, give the bag an ice bath.

5. Meanwhile, make the pickled wild spring onion. Start by combining the sugar, vinegar, and water in a saucepan and place over medium-high flame. Bring to a simmer, stirring constantly, until the sugar is dissolved. Turn off the heat.

6. Rinse and drain the spring onion then place in a bowl. Add the sugar mixture and mix well. Then, chill using an ice bath. Transfer the spring onion mixture into a plastic bag and vacuum seal set to medium. Chill in the refrigerator until ready to serve.

7. To serve, spoon some of the sauce on top of each plate. Then, arrange the sweet onion on top. Drain the wild spring onion and add on top as well. Garnish with chopped chives and Japanese mustard greens, if desired. Serve right away.

Vegetarian Ramen

Total Preparation Time: 3 hours

Temperature: 85 °C (or 185 °F)

Number of Servings: 4

You will need:

- 2 eggs, soft boiled and halved

- 450 grams sweet potatoes, peeled and diced

- 340 grams ramen noodles fresh or cooked

- 225 grams fresh shiitake mushrooms, sliced

- 1 small leek, white only, minced

- 6 garlic cloves, peeled and minced

- 2 ½ cm. piece fresh ginger, peeled and minced

- 1 green onion, sliced thinly

- 16 grams dried shiitake mushrooms

- 3 cups filtered water

- 2 ½ Tbsp. yellow or white miso

- 1 ½ Tbsp. canola oil

- Tamari, as needed

How to prepare:

1. Place the sweet potatoes with a ½ tablespoon of can-ola oil into a plastic bag and seal set to medium-high.

2. Cook the sweet potatoes at the desired temperature level for 1 hour. Then, remove from the hot water and set aside.

3. In a large plastic bag, combine 4 garlic cloves with the ginger, filtered water, white or yellow miso, and dried shiitake mushrooms. Vacuum seal set to medium-low.

4. Cook in the desired temperature level for about 30 minutes. Then, remove from the hot water and set

aside.

5. Place a saucepan over medium-high flame and add the remaining canola oil. Then, sauté the fresh shiitake mushrooms until browned evenly. Transfer to a bowl and set aside to cool slightly.

6. Once slightly cooled, transfer the cooked shiitake mushrooms into a plastic bag and add the yellow onion, garlic cloves, and leek whites. Seal to medium-low.

7. Cook at the desired temperature level for 20 minutes. Then, remove from the hot water and set aside.

8. Set the oven to 400 °F to preheat.

9. Take the sweet potatoes out of the plastic bag and drain. Spread half the sweet potatoes on a baking sheet and bake in the oven for 3 to 5 minutes, or until evenly golden brown. Place the remaining sweet potatoes into a food processor and blend until smooth.

10. Strain the sous vide dried shiitake mushroom mixture and discard the solids. Pour the liquid into a

saucepan and stir in the pureed sweet potatoes. Stir in the cooked shiitake mushroom mixture and bring to a boil. Once boiling, season with tamari to taste.

11. Divide the ramen noodles into 4 servings then ladle the hot broth on top. Half the soft-boiled eggs and place on top of each serving. Top with the roasted sweet potato cubes and serve right away.

7 - Poultry and Seafood Recipes

Chicken Curry Salad

Total Preparation Time: 3 hours 30 minutes

Temperature: 66 °C (or 150 °F)

Number of Servings: 6

You will need:

- 900 grams boneless and skinless chicken breasts

- 330 grams salad greens

- 80 grams toasted chopped walnuts

- 20 grams red curry powder

- 12 red grapes, halved

- ¾ cup high-quality thick mayonnaise

- 1/3 tsp. Worcestershire sauce

How to prepare:

1. Rinse the chicken breasts then blot dry with paper towels. Season the chicken breasts with a bit of the curry powder then place them in a plastic bag and

seal set to medium-low.

2. Cook at the desired room temperature level for 1 hour, then transfer to an ice bath and chill before transferring to the refrigerator. Chill for at least 2 hours.

3. Once chilled, dice the chicken breasts into bite-sized pieces and place in a bowl. Add the walnut, red grapes, remaining curry powder, mayonnaise, and Worcestershire sauce. Toss to combine.

4. Divide the salad greens into individual servings and heap the chicken curry salad on top of each. Serve right away.

Sous Vide Fried Chicken

Total Preparation Time: 3 hours

Temperature: 68 °C (or 155 °F) and 63 °C (or 145 °F)

Number of Servings: 6

You will need:

- 1.7 kilograms whole chicken

- 375 grams all-purpose flour

- 354 milliliters buttermilk

- 20 grams dried tarragon

- 0.5 grams garlic powder

- 0.5 grams smoked paprika

- 0.25 grams onion powder

- Peanut oil, as needed

How to prepare:

1. Have the shop chop up the chicken into 12 equal pieces. Have the bones pulled out of the breast halves. Rinse the chicken pieces then blot dry with paper towels. Set aside.

2. In a bowl, mix together the garlic and onion powders, tarragon, and smoked paprika. Season the chicken pieces all over with the spice mixture then place the wings and halved breasts together in one bag and the remaining pieces in another bag. Seal set to medium-low.

3. Cook the chicken thighs, legs and other parts in 68 °C (or 155 °F) for 1 hour. Then, reduce to 63 °C (or 145 °F) and add the bag of chicken wings and breast. Cook for an additional hour. Transfer the bags into an ice bath.

4. Once chilled, remove the chicken pieces from the plastic bags and season all over with sea salt. Prepare the buttermilk in one pan and the all-purpose flour in another.

5. Coat the chicken pieces in the flour then dip in the buttermilk. Then, dip in the flour once again. Set aside for 15 minutes at room temperature.

6. Meanwhile, pour about 8 cups of peanut oil into a heavy duty pot and heat over a high flame to 204 °C (or 400 °F).

7. Once the oil is ready, add the chicken pieces and cook for 2 minutes or until golden brown. Transfer the fried chicken to a pan lined with paper towels and drain. Best served freshly cooked.

Hearty Chicken, Vegetable, And Egg Noodle Soup

Total Preparation Time: 3 hours

Temperature: 84 °C (or 183 °F) for the vegetables and 64 °C (or 147 °F) for the chicken

Number of Servings: 4

You will need:

- 450 grams fresh baby spinach

- 170 grams boneless and skinless chicken breasts, diced

- 75 grams dried egg noodles

- 30 grams diced white onion

- 30 grams diced yellow squash

- 30 grams diced red bell pepper

- 15 grams diced carrot

- 1 liter chicken broth

- ½ Tbsp. extra virgin olive oil

- 2 grams garlic powder

- 2 grams onion powder

- Sea salt, as needed

- Freshly ground black pepper, as needed

How to prepare:

1. Combine the carrot, red bell pepper, yellow squash, baby spinach, and white onion in a mixing bowl. Drizzle in the olive oil and turn gently to coat.

2. Sprinkle with the garlic and onion powders followed by a pinch of sea salt and black pepper. Toss well to coat.

3. Transfer the vegetables to a plastic bag and seal set to medium-high. Then, cook at the desired temperature level for 1 hour. Then, remove from the hot bath and place in an ice bath. Then, transfer to the refrigerator and chill until ready to serve.

4. Meanwhile, set the sous vide machine to the desired temperature level for the chicken.

5. Place the chicken breasts in a plastic bag and seal set to medium. Then, cook for 1 hour at the desired temperature level. Remove from the heat and set aside.

6. Pour the chicken broth into a pot. Strain the liquids from the vegetables and chicken and pour into the pot. Bring to a boil over a high flame then add the egg noodles. Cook according to the package instructions.

7. Stir in the vegetables and chicken into the broth and reduce to low flame. Cook until the vegetables and chicken are heated through. Then, ladle into bowls and serve right away.

Coq Au Vin

Total Preparation Time: 5 hours

Temperature: 64 °C (or 147 °F)

Number of Servings: 6

You will need:

- 3 kilograms whole chickens, chopped, breastbones removed

- 150 grams Italian plum tomatoes

- 3 white onions, diced

- 3 garlic cloves, peeled and minced

- 225 grams sliced fresh white button mushrooms

- 355 milliliters pinot noir

- 355 milliliters chicken stock

- 4 ½ Tbsp. extra virgin olive oil

- 2 bay leaves

- 1.5 grams dried thyme

- Sea salt, as needed

- Freshly ground black pepper, as needed

How to prepare:

1. Rinse the chicken pieces thoroughly then blot dry with paper towels. Season all over with sea salt.

2. Place a sauté pan over medium high flame and add the olive oil. Add the chicken and sear for 3 minutes per side. Transfer to a plate and let cool for 15

minutes.

3. Meanwhile, sauté the white onion and white button mushrooms in the same pan, then add the garlic and sauté until everything is heated through and browned.

4. Add the pinot noir and stir, scraping the browned bits on the pan. Increase to high flame and boil until the liquid is reduced by half. Then, stir in the tomato, thyme, bay leaf, and chicken stock. Bring to a boil and continue until the liquid is again reduced by half.

5. Turn off the heat and allow the temperature to cool slightly, then transfer to a bowl, cover, and chill for 30 minutes in the refrigerator.

6. Place the seared chicken into a plastic bag and add the chilled liquids. Then, seal set to medium-low.

7. Cook the chicken at the desired temperature level for 3 hours, and then remove from the hot water.

8. Transfer the chicken and sauce out of the bag and re-move the bay leaf. Then, season to taste with salt and pepper and divide into individual servings. This is

best served right away.

John Dory And Sea Scallops With Asparagus And Mousseline Sauce

Total Preparation Time: 1 hour

Temperature: 60 °C (or 140 °F) for the John Dory and Sea Scallops and 85 °C (or 185 °F) for the Asparagus

Number of Servings: 6

You will need:

- 3 kilograms John Dory, skins removed

- 115 grams sea scallops, muscles removed

- 120 grams crème fraiche

- 42 grams heavy cream

- Sea salt, to taste

For the Asparagus:

- 18 medium asparagus spears

- 75 grams cold milk

- 25 grams water

- Granulated sugar, as needed

- Sea salt, to taste

For the Mousseline Sauce:

- 2 medium egg yolks

- ½ small lemon

- 128 grams clarified butter, melted and kept warm

- 96 grams champagne vinegar

- 30 grams whipped cream

- 20 grams water

- 15 grams thinly sliced shallots

- 2 fresh tarragon sprigs

- 5 black peppercorns

How to prepare:

1. Fillet the John Dory, slicing off the belly and saving it. Separate the fillets to get six equal pieces. Trim the

pieces into rectangles to create approximately 80 grams each. Refrigerate the fillets.

2. Meanwhile, combine the belly with the scallops and crème fraiche in a food processor. Process until smooth then add the cream gradually as you process.

3. Transfer the mixture to a metal bowl and place the bowl into a bowl of ice water. Season with salt and transfer to a refrigerator. Refrigerate until chilled.

4. Once the fish fillets are chilled, season them with salt and then set aside for 3 minutes. After that, blot dry with paper towels and arrange in a single layer in a large plastic bag. Spoon the pureed seafood mixture on top of the fish fillets and spread. Then, vacuum pack on low.

5. Cook at the desired temperature level for 10 minutes.

6. To prepare the asparagus, snap off the tough ends then peel them and trim the ends to ensure all the spears are of equal length.

7. Place the spears in a plastic bag in a single layer with the tips facing upward. Sprinkle in the granulated

sugar and salt then pour in the milk. Vacuum seal set to medium-high.

8. Cook the asparagus spears at the desired temperature level for 30 minutes or until tender. Then transfer to an ice bath.

9. To prepare the mousseline sauce, mix together the shallot, vinegar, peppercorns, and tarragon in a saucepan. Place over medium flame and simmer until mixture turns syrupy. Then, add the water and stir to combine.

10. Strain the mixture into a bowl and pour half into a saucepan. Add the egg yolks and whisk over the lowest possible heat setting for about 2 minutes. Remove the pan from the heat and then gradually add the butter as you continue to stir. Make sure the sauce becomes thickened before you add more butter.

11. Once thickened, stir in the lemon juice and season with salt. Add the whipped cream and fold to combine.

12. Divide the mousseline sauce among the serving dishes, followed by the fish fillets and asparagus

spears. Serve right away.

Poached Tuna With Eggplant, Olives, Tomatoes, And Pine Nuts

Total Preparation Time: 30 minutes

Temperature: 59.5 °C (or 139.1 °F)

Number of Servings: 6

You will need:

- 2 medium Italian eggplants

- 18 Niçoise olives, pitted and sliced

- 330 grams Atlantic Bluefin tuna, top loin, cold

- 225 grams heirloom tomatoes, peeled and chopped

- 60 grams extra virgin olive oil

- 60 grams canola oil

- 15 grams pine nuts

- 375 milligrams organic basil seeds

- Extra virgin olive oil, as needed

- Balsamic vinegar, as needed

- Sea salt, as needed

How to prepare:

1. Put the basil seeds into a bowl along with about 375 grams of room temperature water. Set aside to soak for 1 hour.

2. Slice the eggplants into thin rounds and set aside. Place a skillet over medium flame and add enough olive oil to coat. Swirl to coat then cook the eggplant until warmed through, but not browned. Transfer to a plate lined with paper towels and season with salt.

3. In a nonstick skillet, add just enough olive oil to coat and place over medium-low flame. Once hot, stir in the pine nuts and cook until toasted and fragrant. Drain and place on a plate lined with paper towels. Season lightly with salt.

4. Drizzle the tomatoes with olive oil and balsamic vinegar. Then, add the eggplant and olives and toss well to combine.

5. Drain the basil seeds and set aside.

6. Place the tuna inside a bag and pour in the canola and extra virgin olive oils. Vacuum seal set to medium.

7. Cook the tuna at the desired temperature level for 13 minutes. Then, transfer the tuna onto a rack placed over a tray and set aside to drain.

8. Once drained, slice the tuna into 1-inch cubes and lightly coat with olive oil. Divide the eggplant and tomato mixture among six servings and add the tuna on top. Sprinkle with the pine nuts and basil seeds then serve right away.

Halibut With Black-Eyed Pea And Bacon Salad

Total Preparation Time: x hours

Temperature: 62 °C (or 143.6 °F)

Number of Servings: 6

You will need:

- 3 halibut bellies, about 350 grams per piece

- 3 large eggs

- 195 grams Dijon mustard

- 188 grams fresh breadcrumbs

- 16 grams pureed roasted garlic

- 3 grams minced fresh flat leaf parsley

- Sea salt, to taste

- Freshly ground black pepper, to taste

- Clarified butter, as needed

For the black-eyed peas:

- 315 grams fresh black-eyed peas

- 700 grams chicken stock

- 700 grams water

- 218 grams bacon, chopped into six strips

- 90 grams peeled onion

- 80 grams peeled, seeded and diced tomatoes

- 75 grams carrot

- 53 grams leek, light green and white parts

- 65 grams unsalted butter

- 5 grams minced shallot

- 1.5 grams minced fresh flat leaf parsley

- 3 fresh thyme sprigs

- Champagne vinegar, as needed

- Sea salt, as needed

How to prepare:

1. Trim the halibut bellies then slice in half crosswise. Season with salt all over and set aside for 10 minutes. Then, blot dry with paper towels.

2. Place the halibut bellies into plastic bags in a single layer and vacuum seal on medium. Cook at the desired temperature level for 11 minutes, then transfer to an ice bath to chill. Once chilled, remove the bellies and set aside on a plate lined with paper towels.

3. Meanwhile, beat the eggs, Dijon mustard, and pureed roasted garlic in a bowl. On a plate, combine the

breadcrumbs, parsley, and add a pinch of salt and pepper. Mix well.

4. Preheat the oven to 350 degrees F.

5. Dip each fillet in the egg, and then dredge in the crumb mixture. Repeat and then tap off the excess. Once all the fillets are coated, coat an ovenproof pan with clarified butter and arrange the coated fillets on it in a single layer. Bake for 5 minutes, then flip over and back for an additional 5 minutes.

6. To prepare the black-eyed peas, pour them into a pot and add the water, chicken stock, onion, carrot, and bacon.

7. Halve the leek lengthwise and rinse well in cold running water. Stuff the parsley and thyme sprigs between the leek and then tie with butcher's twine to secure. Add the leek to the pot.

8. Place the pot over a medium-high flame and simmer. Continue to simmer for 15 to 20 minutes, or until the peas are tender. After that, remove from the heat and set aside to cool to room temperature.

9. Once cooled, remove the carrot, leek, and onion from the pot and strain the peas using a fine mesh strainer, saving the liquids into a saucepan. Transfer the black-eyed peas to a bowl and set aside.

10. Heat the liquids over medium flame until reduced, then add the peas and bring to a boil. Stir in the butter and let simmer until the mixture is creamy. Finally, stir in the tomato, shallot, and parsley. Season to taste with salt and champagne vinegar.

11. To serve, divide the fillets into individual servings and top with the black-eyed peas. Serve right away.

Savory Squid And Heart Of Palm With Lemon Seafood Vinaigrette

Total Preparation Time: 10 hours and 30 minutes

Temperature: 64 °C (or 147.2 °F)

Number of Servings: 9

You will need:

- 2 kilograms fresh squid

- 30 grams extra virgin olive oil

- 1.5 grams cumin seeds

- 1.5 grams coriander seeds

- 3 dried red chilies

- 2 fresh thyme sprigs

- 2 rosemary sprigs

- 3 bay leaves

- Sea salt, as needed

- Freshly ground black pepper, as needed

For the heart of palm:

- 1200 grams fresh heart of palm

- Sea salt, as needed

- Extra virgin olive oil, as needed

For the seafood lemon vinaigrette:

- 60 grams canola oil

- 30 grams lemon oil

- 30 grams strained squid ink

- 7.5 grams Dijon mustard

- 2 pieces freshly peeled lemon zest

How to prepare:

1. Carefully twist the head from the squid and then pull it away from its body. Carefully puncture the ink sac and save its ink into a bowl.

2. Then, slice the tentacles away from the head. Remove and discard the entrails and eyes then remove the beak from the middle of the tentacles. Then, remove the cuttlebone from the body.

3. Slice the body open lengthwise then spread it open. Lay on a chopping board with the inner side facing up. Then, refrigerate until chilled.

4. Meanwhile, place the ink into a saucepan and heat over medium flame, whisking throughout, until slightly thickened. Then, whisk in the Dijon mustard followed by the canola oil and lemon oil. Finally, add the lemon zest and mix well. Cover and refrigerate until ready to serve.

5. Combine the coriander and cumin seeds, red chilies, thyme, rosemary, and bay leaves into a tea bag.

6. Once the squid is chilled, place it in a plastic bag with the bag of herbs and spices. Add the olive oil and a pinch of salt and pepper. Then, vacuum seal set to medium.

7. Cook the squid at the desired temperature level for 10 hours. Then, place the bag in an ice bath. Once chilled, remove the squid from the bag and cut cross-wise into thin strips. Set aside in a bowl.

8. Prepare the heart of palm by slicing it into extra thin strips. Separate the heart of palm strips and then place them in a bowl. Add the squid strips and toss to combine. Add a drizzle of olive oil and a pinch of salt to taste and toss well to combine.

9. Drizzle the vinaigrette on the serving dish and heat the squid and heart of palm strips on top. Serve right away.

8 - Red Meat Recipes

Beef Tenderloin With Caramelized Garlic

Total Preparation Time: 45 minutes

Temperature: 66 °C (or 150 °F)

Number of Servings: 8

You will need:

- 1.8 kilograms beef tenderloin

- 3 garlic cloves, crushed and peeled

- 3 fresh thyme sprigs

- 112 grams unsalted butter

- Canola oil, as needed

- Sea salt, as needed

- Freshly ground black pepper, as needed

For the Caramelized Garlic:

- 9 garlic cloves, peeled and halved

- Granulated sugar, as needed

How to prepare:

1. Trim off the fat and sinew from the beef tenderloin then season all over with salt and pepper. Set aside for 10 minutes.

2. After 10 minutes, blot the tenderloin with paper towels and place in a plastic bag. Vacuum seal set to medium and refrigerate for about 6 hours.

3. After chilling, cook the bag of tenderloin in the desired temperature level for 40 minutes.

4. Meanwhile, prepare the garlic by placing them in a saucepan and adding enough cold water to cover. Place over medium flame and heat until boiling. Once boiling, drain and place the garlic back into the saucepan. Add more cold water to cover and bring to a boil. Continue to boil until the garlic is tender, and then drain.

5. Add about 25 grams of water into the saucepan with the garlic then sprinkle in about a pinch of sugar. Simmer until the water is evaporated and the garlic is golden brown and caramelized. Set aside.

6. Once the beef tenderloin is ready, place a cast iron skillet over medium-high flame and add enough canola oil to coat. Heat until smoking. Drain the tenderloin and blot dry, then place into the hot oil and sear for 7 minutes.

7. Stir the butter, garlic, and thyme into the skillet and cook the tenderloin around it. Then, transfer the meat to a plate and let rest for 10 minutes.

8. Slice the tenderloin against the grain and divide into separate servings. Add the caramelized garlic on the side and serve right away.

Hearty Beef And Barley Stew

Total Preparation Time: 18 hours

Temperature: 66 °C (or 150 °F) and 88 °C (or 190 °F)

Number of Servings: 6

You will need:

- ¾ kilograms beef stew meat, sliced into ½-inch cubes

- 1 liter beef stock

- 14 milliliters Worcestershire sauce

- 200 grams diced celery

- 200 grams diced white onion

- 200 grams diced carrots

- 170 grams uncooked barley

- 7 grams chopped tarragon

- Freshly ground black pepper, as needed

How to prepare:

1. Rinse the beef stew meat thoroughly then blot dry with paper towels. Season with black pepper and place in a plastic bag. Vacuum seal set to medium.

2. Cook the beef at the desired temperature level for 16 hours.

3. Remove the bag of beef from the hot water and set the temperature to 88 °C (or 190 °F). Place the bag of beef into an ice bath.

4. Pour the beef broth into a plastic bag and add Worcestershire sauce, white onion, celery, and barley. Vacuum seal set to low then cook at the desired temperature for 1 hour.

5. Once the barley is ready, transfer the contents into a pot along with the beef. Place over high heat and simmer until heated through. Ladle into soup bowls and serve right away.

Rosemary Beef Spare Ribs

Total Preparation Time: 73 hours

Temperature: 54 °C (or 130 °F)

Number of Servings: 6

You will need:

- 3 kilograms beef spare ribs

- 1 Tbsp. chopped fresh rosemary leaves

- Sea salt, as needed

- Granulated sugar, as needed

- Freshly ground black pepper, as needed

How to prepare:

1. Trim off the excess fat from the beef spare ribs. Sprinkle the sea salt, sugar, black pepper, and rosemary all over the ribs, then place in a plastic bag. Vacuum seal set to medium.

2. Cook the beef at the desired temperature level for 72 hours. At the end of the cooking time, take the plastic bag out of the water and then remove the spare ribs. Blot the spare ribs dry with paper towels.

3. Strain the liquid into a saucepan and place over a high flame. Simmer into a glaze then set aside.

4. Scrape the meat from the bones and sear the meat in a preheated cast iron skillet or grill to form a crust, about 1 minute per side.

5. Place the meat on a platter and spoon the glaze on top. Serve right away.

Lamb Saddle With Garden Vegetables And Traditional Hot Italian Sauce

Total Preparation Time: 1 hour

Temperature: 60.5 °C (or 140.9 °F)

Number of Servings: 8

You will need:

- 2 lamb saddles, split bone-in with flank attached

- 100 grams unsalted butter

- 30 grams extra virgin olive oil

- 4 garlic cloves, crushed and peeled

- 4 fresh thyme sprigs

- Canola oil, as needed

- Sea salt, as needed

- Freshly ground black pepper, as needed

For the Vegetables:

- 50 grams, chopped carrot

- 50 grams chopped cauliflower florets

- 50 grams chopped red bell pepper

- 50 grams chopped yellow bell pepper

- 50 grams chopped artichoke thistle

- 50 grams chopped fennel

- Canola oil, as needed

- Sea salt, as needed

- Freshly ground black pepper, as needed

For the Sauce:

- 1 lemon

- 1000 grams lamb stock

- 1000 grams beef stock

- 100 grams unsalted butter

- 76 grams red wine vinegar

- 50 grams extra virgin olive oil

- 40 grams pureed roasted garlic

- 30 grams minced shallot

- 20 grams minced garlic

- 20 grams chopped fresh flat leaf parsley

- 16 grams anchovy packed in salt, rinsed

- Canola oil, as needed

- Sea salt, as needed

How to prepare:

1. Place a cast iron skillet over medium flame and add enough canola oil to coat. Halve the lemon and place the cut sides down. Cook until caramelized for 30 minutes, swirling occasionally. Set aside.

2. In a saucepan over medium flame, heat 30 grams of the olive oil. Sauté the shallot, garlic, parsley and a pinch of salt. Sauté for 3 minutes then stir in the vinegar. Sauté for 3 minutes, then add the anchovy and sauté, breaking down the anchovy, until the vinegar is dried off.

3. Pour the stocks into the anchovy mixture and bring to a simmer. Continue to simmer for 20 minutes, then

strain into a bowl. Discard the solids.

4. Return the liquid into a saucepan and stir in the lemon halves. Then, simmer for 1 hour or until the mixture turns into a light sauce. Stir in the pureed roasted garlic, butter, remaining olive oil, and lemon zest. Season to taste with salt.

5. To prepare the lamb saddle, bone and remove the loin and tenderloin. Slice the flank from the fat but ensure the fat is still attached to the loin. Set the flank aside for another dish. Trim off the silver skin and trim the fat. Score the outside of the fat. Season the tenderloin and loin all over with salt and pepper. Add the tenderloin on top.

6. Roll the lamb to even out the meat and then tie securely with butcher's twine. Refrigerate for 6 hours.

7. Place the garlic cloves and 2 thyme sprigs into a tea bag. Place the lamb in a plastic bag and add the olive oil and bag of garlic and thyme. Vacuum seal set to medium.

8. Cook at the desired temperature level for 40 minutes, then take the lamb out of the bag and blot dry with

paper towels. Season with salt and pepper.

9. Place a cast iron skillet over medium-high flame and add a film of canola oil. Cook for 3 minutes or until browned all over.

10. Drain the oils from the skillet save for 50 grams. Reduce to medium flame and place the butter and remaining thyme sprigs into the skillet. Cook, basting the lamb with the butter, for about 3 minutes.

11. Place the lamb on a rack and let rest for 10 minutes, then slice into 8 medallions.

12. To prepare the vegetables, place a skillet over medium flame and add a coat of canola oil. Stir fry the carrot, cauliflower, fennel, bell peppers, and artichoke thistle until crisp and tender. Season to taste with salt and pepper.

13. To serve, spoon the sauce on top of each dish and divide the vegetables among them. Place the medallion of lamb on top and serve right away.

Korean Inspired Short Ribs

Total Preparation Time: 49 hours

8 - RED MEAT RECIPES

Temperature: 60 °C (or 140 °F)

Number of Servings: 6

You will need:

- 3 kilograms beef spare ribs

- 2 Asian pears, peeled, cored and chopped

- 2 large yellow onions, peeled and chopped

- 600 milliliters filtered water

- 240 milliliters tamari

- 80 milliliters organic apple juice

- 80 milliliters vegetable oil

- 67 milliliters mirin

- 18 milliliters sesame oil

- 1 ½ tsp. ground white pepper

How to prepare:

1. Combine the filtered water, apple juice, mirin, tamari, sesame oil, white pepper, yellow onions, and

Asian pears in a food processor and blend into a slurry.

2. Pour the mixture into two plastic bags and divide the beef spare ribs between them. Turn several times to coat then vacuum seal on medium.

3. Cook the spare ribs for 48 hours at the desired temperature level.

4. At the end of the cooking time, take the spare ribs out of the hot water and set aside. Take the ribs out of the bag and place on a platter. Strain the liquids into a saucepan.

5. Place the saucepan with the liquids over a high flame and simmer until the liquid is reduced to 3 cups. Set aside.

6. Scrape the meat from the bones of the spare ribs and set aside.

7. Place a cast iron skillet over medium-high flame and add the vegetable oil. Add the meat and cook for 4 minutes per side, or until a deep brown color.

8. Take the short ribs out of the skillet and pour the

sauce on top. Serve right away.

Beef Sirloin With Bone Marrow Sauce

Total Preparation Time: 1 hour and 15 minutes

Temperature: 59.5 °C (or 139.1 °F)

Number of Servings: 6

You will need:

- 600 grams prime beef sirloin, cold

- 24 grams unsalted butter

- 3 garlic cloves, peeled

- 2 fresh thyme sprigs

- Sea salt, as needed

- Freshly ground black pepper, as needed

- Canola oil, as needed

For the Bone Marrow Sauce:

- 750 grams beef stock

- 80 grams rendered bone marrow fat, warm

- 45 grams crème fraiche

- 15 grams minced shallot

- 8 black peppercorns

- 2 fresh thyme sprigs

- Champagne vinegar, as needed

- Sea salt, as needed

How to prepare:

1. Season the beef sirloin all over with salt and pepper, then place inside a bag and vacuum seal set to medium.

2. Cook the sirloin for 1 hour at the desired temperature. Then, remove from the hot water and set aside for 10 minutes.

3. After 10 minutes, place a cast iron skillet over medium flame and add enough canola oil to coat. Once hot, add the beef sirloin and cook for 5 minutes or until browned all over.

4. Add the garlic, thyme, and butter to the skillet with the sirloin and turn over the meat. Make sure to tilt the skillet and spoon the butter over the sirloin as you cook.

5. Transfer the sirloin to a platter and let rest for 10 minutes.

6. Meanwhile, prepare the bone marrow sauce by combining the stock with the shallot, thyme, and peppercorn in a saucepan. Place over medium-high flame and bring to a simmer. Reduce to medium flame and continue to simmer until the liquid is reduced.

7. Strain the stock mixture into a blender and add the crème fraiche. Pulse the mixture to combine. Continue to pulse as you gradually pour into the warm bone marrow fat. Then, add a sprinkle of vinegar and a pinch of salt. Blend and pour back into the saucepan. Heat over a low flame.

8. To serve, spoon the bone marrow sauce onto each serving dish. Slice the beef sirloin across the grain thinly and lay on top of the plate. Serve right away.

9 - Dessert Recipes

Banana Sherbet

Total Preparation Time: 1 hour

Temperature: 85 °C (or 185 °F)

Number of Servings: 15

You will need:

- 6 firm bananas

- 480 grams pure maple syrup

- 180 grams whole milk

- 1.5 kilograms freshly squeezed orange juice

- 338 grams granulated sugar

- 1 ½ vanilla beans, split

How to prepare:

1. Pour the sugar into a saucepan and place over medium flame. Heat until the sugar is caramelized then reduce to low flame and stir in the vanilla seeds and pod. Stir in the orange juice until the mixture is com-

bined.

2. Strain the mixture and pour into a heatproof bowl. Then place over an ice bath and then transfer into the refrigerator to chill.

3. Once the sugar mixture is chilled, peel the bananas and place into a plastic bag. Add the chilled sugar mixture and then turn several times to coat the bananas in the mixture.

4. Fold the bag firmly around the bananas and vacuum seal set to medium.

5. Then, cook at the desired temperature level for 45 minutes, or until the bananas become extra tender.

6. Transfer the mixture to a food processor and blend until smooth and thick. Pour in the milk and blend again until smooth. Pour into a container and chill in the ice bath. Transfer to an ice cream maker and freeze according to manufacturer's instructions. Best served chilled.

Braised Golden Pineapple

Total Preparation Time: 1 hour and 20 minutes

Temperature: 75 °C (or 167 °F)

Number of Servings: 8 to 12

You will need:

- 2.25 kilograms under-ripe pineapple

- 325 grams granulated sugar

- 1 ½ vanilla beans, split

- 400 milliliters dry white wine

- 400 milliliters water

- 400 milliliters granulated sugar

How to prepare:

1. Combine the dry white wine with the water and 400 milliliters granulated sugar in a bowl and set aside.

2. Slice off both ends of the pineapple then peel off the skin. Set it up to stand on one end, then slice the pineapple vertically to expose the core. Slice the pineapple pieces into big rectangles then set aside.

3. In a saucepan, mix together the vanilla beans and

sugar then place over medium flame. Cook until cara-melized then reduce to low flame and cook, stirring frequently, until the mixture becomes a golden brown caramel.

4. Pour the wine and sugar mixture into the saucepan and stir well to combine. Then, add the sliced pine-apple and simmer for 6 minutes, turning the pine-apples halfway through to coat.

5. Place the pineapple slices onto a platter and let cool slightly, then cover with a plastic wrap and store in the freezer for about 3 hours until completely cooled.

6. Meanwhile, strain the caramel into a bowl and place in an ice bath to chill. Then, transfer to the refriger-ator to continue to chill.

7. Once the pineapple and caramel are completely chilled, divide them into bags, making sure the pine-apples are laid in a single layer and coated in the car-amel.

8. Vacuum seal the pineapples set to medium, then cook at the desired temperature level for 1 hour. Then, transfer to an ice bath and refrigerate.

9. To serve, remove the pineapple from the bag and transfer to a plate. If desired, slice into artful shapes and arrange on a plate. Spoon the syrup on top then serve chilled.

Cherry Ice Cream

Total Preparation Time: 30 minutes

Temperature: 85 °C (or 185 °F)

Number of Servings: 15

You will need:

- 8 medium egg yolks

- 562.5 grams pureed Bing cherries

- 562.5 grams pureed sour cherries

- 375 grams 40 percent heavy cream

- 375 grams whole milk

- 196 grams pure maple syrup

- 46 grams granulated sugar

- 46 grams liquid glucose

How to prepare:

1. Mix together the pureed cherries in a saucepan and place over medium flame. Simmer until the mixture is reduced by half. Turn off the heat and stir in the milk and cream, then strain into a bowl and set aside.

2. In a stand mixer, beat the egg yolks together with the liquid glucose and sugar until the eggs are pale yellow and form into thin ribbons. Mix in the pureed cherry then strain into a bowl.

3. Refrigerate the mixture for at least 3 hours or until chilled. Then, transfer into a bag and vacuum seal set to medium.

4. Heat the water to the desired temperature level then add the bag. After that, set the temperature to 82 °C (or 179.6°F) and cook for 25 minutes.

5. Remove the bag from the hot water and then lay it on a flat surface. Tilt the bag slightly to mix well and let stand for 5 minutes at room temperature. Then, transfer into an ice bath.

6. Transfer the bag to the refrigerator for 6 hours, then strain and fold in the maple syrup. Transfer to an ice cream machine and prepare according to the manufacturer's instructions. Best served chilled.

Cashew Ice Cream

Total Preparation Time: 1 hour

Temperature: 85 °C (or 185 °F)

Number of Servings: 12

You will need:

- 10 large egg yolks

- 750 grams whole milk

- 500 grams raw unsalted cashews

- 250 grams 32 percent heavy cream

- 187 grams pure maple syrup

- 40 grams atomized glucose

- 50 grams granulated sugar

- 50 grams dry milk powder

- Canola oil, as needed

How to prepare:

1. Set the oven to 300 °F to preheat.

2. Spread the unsalted cashews on a baking sheet and then roast for 5 minutes. Then, remove from the oven and place into the food processor. Blend until the cashews turn into a pasty consistency.

3. Pour a bit of canola oil into the food processor with the cashews and blend until smooth. Strain the cashew mixture into a bowl and set aside.

4. Meanwhile, beat the egg yolks and sugar in a stand mixer and blend until the egg yolks turn pale yellow and fall into ribbons when poured. Set aside.

5. Pour the milk and cream into a saucepan and place over lowest possible setting. Heat until just warm, then stir in the dry milk powder and glucose. Mix well.

6. Set the stand mixer with the egg yolks to low speed

and gradually pour in the cream mixture. Mix well, then strain again into a bowl. Cover and refrigerate until cold.

7. Once cold, pour the yolk mixture into a plastic bag and vacuum seal set to medium until the mixture becomes bubbly.

8. Preheat the sous vide cooker to the desired temperature level, then add the bag. Then, reduce to 82°C (or 179.6 °F). Cook for 30 minutes.

9. Remove the bag from the hot water and then lay it on a flat surface. Tilt the bag slightly to mix well and let stand for 5 minutes at room temperature. Then, transfer into a bowl and fold in the cashew paste. Chill in an ice bath and then cover and refrigerate for 12 to 24 hours.

10. Strain the mixture then transfer to an ice cream machine and prepare according to the manufacturer's instructions. Best served chilled.

Candied Apple Balls And Ginger Custard

Total Preparation Time: 2 hours

Temperature: 85 °C (or 185 °F) for the Ginger Custard and 75 °C (or 167 °F) for the Candied Applies

Number of Servings: 6 to 8

You will need:

For the Candied Apples:

- 6 Golden Delicious apples

- 400 milliliters dry white wine

- 400 milliliters water

- 400 milliliters granulated sugar

For the Ginger Custard

- 5 large egg yolks

- 325 grams 40 percent heavy cream

- 250 grams whole milk

- 62 grams granulated sugar

- 50 grams freshly peeled ginger

- 2.5 grams powdered ginger

- 1 gram gelatin sheet, soaked in cold water

- Sea salt, as needed

How to prepare:

1. Mix together the dry white wine, water, and granulated sugar into a saucepan. Place over a high flame and bring to a boil, stirring constantly until the sugar is dissolved. Turn off the heat and let cool to room temperature. Then, transfer to the refrigerator and chill.

2. Peel the apples and use a melon baller to scoop into balls. Arrange the balls into a plastic bag in a single layer then pour in the chilled sugar mixture. Vacuum seal set to medium and refrigerate until chilled.

3. Once chilled, cook the apple balls at the desired temperature level for 1 hour and 30 minutes, or until the apples are candied. Transfer to an ice bath and keep chilled until ready to serve.

4. To prepare the ginger custard, heat 250 grams of the cream and the milk in a saucepan over low flame; do not bring to a simmer.

5. Crush the ginger and stir into the mixture followed by the powdered ginger. Mix well then remove from heat and cover. Set aside for 10 minutes.

6. After steeping the mixture, strain and discard the solids.

7. In a stand mixer, beat the yolks together with the sugar and a dash of salt until pale yellow and the mixture turns into a fine ribbon. Then, set to low speed and blend in the ginger cream mixture until combined.

8. Strain the mixture into a bowl and then chill in an ice bath. Once chilled, transfer into a plastic bag and vacuum seal set to medium.

9. Heat the water to the desired temperature level then reduce the heat to 82 °C (or 179.6 °F). Cook for 10 minutes.

10. After 10 minutes, tilt the bag slightly to combine the mixture again. Then set aside for 5 minutes at room temperature.

11. Transfer the custard to a bowl. Press the excess water

from the gelatin sheet and stir it into the custard. Strain again and pour the custard into a bowl. Place in an ice bath to chill.

12. Beat the remaining cream until soft peaks form. Gradually fold the whipped cream into the custard then transfer into a bowl and refrigerate until set and ready to serve.

13. To serve, place the candied apple balls on a serving platter and spoon the ginger custard on the side. Serve right away.

10 - Conclusion

Now that you have reached the end of this book, it is safe to say that you have learned how to do sous vide confidently in your kitchen. There are plenty of other wonderful recipes out there that you can try. You can also experiment with your own versions of these recipes for added variety.

There is no limit to the number of dishes you can make, and at this point, you know that if you want the best flavor, texture, and quality of food, you should not hesitate to cook sous vide.

Book 3 - Sous Vide

Modern Techniques for Perfect Cooking Through Science
(Scrumptious Dinners, Gourmet Cookbook, Precision Cooking)

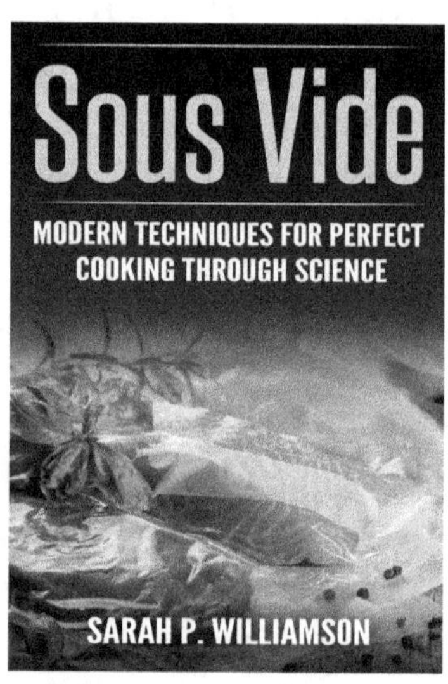

1 - Introduction

Benefits of Cooking the Sous Vide Way

Sous vide sounds too fancy to apply to cooking, but it simply means placing your ingredients in a container (a cooking pouch or canning jar can be used) and then dropping the container into a heated water bath set at a target temperature. As soon as your food reaches the intended time or temperature, you remove it from the water bath, finish (for example, by giving it a quick sear) it, and enjoy it.

Everything Tastes Better

Cooking the sous vide way gives you food that simply tastes way better than if you cooked it using conventional methods. Your tenderloin steaks turn out juicier and perfectly done around the edges, your beef or lamb ribs almost melt as they touch your mouth, your fish fillets are succulent and their centers are as evenly cooked as their edges.

Even an egg can be cooked the sous vide way, and you will be amazed at how delicate and custard-like your poached egg turns out.

Carved in History

Since the ancient times, the practice of preserving and cooking different kinds of food in sealed containers or packages has been around. Culinary history records will tell you that people have been wrapping food in leaves, sealing them inside the bladders of animals, packing them in salt, or potting them in fat prior to cooking.

They already had the idea that preventing food from being exposed to air can slow down its decay - something that vacuum sealing successfully does. As a bonus, packaging your food also helps keep it succulent, not dried out.

Precision, Perfection

"Sous vide" is a French term that means "under vacuum." The sous vide cooking method does utilize vacuum sealing food, but its important feature is precise temperature control. Cooking your food the sous vide way means you use a heater that is computer-controlled to bring a water bath to the target temperature and then keep the water bath at that temperature for hours or days.

Having the ability to control temperature or heat in cooking your food gives you the freedom to go about the cooking process without being a slave to time.

When using the conventional oven or grill, you have to deal with extreme temperatures as well as fluctuating temperatures – this is why it is important to get your exact cooking times straight, since going a little off the mark results in foods that do not turn out as they should.

But if you cook using the sous vide method, your foods are guaranteed to taste just right, giving you ample time to focus on the other aspects of food preparation.

But First, Safety

The sous vide way of cooking's use of accurate and uniform temperatures provide you other benefits:

Your food turn out evenly cooked through, so you can say goodbye to rare centers and overly dried-out edges; you get the same perfectly cooked results every single time you cook; and most importantly, you can rest assured that any potential pathogens in your food, especially in chicken and other poultry meats, are killed for your safety.

Have It All

Lastly, cooking your food in a closed container allows you to provide a completely humid environment for your ingredients. This is what braises your food in an effective manner and gives you markedly more scrumptious and more succulent results.

Simply searing your sous vide cooked food (which do not brown) will give them those traditional flavors you have gotten used to, so you actually get to enjoy both the nostalgic taste of your old style cooking and the gourmet flavors imparted by the scientific sous vide method.

Tips and Tricks for Sous Vide Cooking

Digging into gourmet quality dishes does not have to be tricky. Simplify sous vide cooking by following these tips:

Pouching

Prepping your food for sous vide cooking is as easy as buy, portion, and seal:

1. Purchase economy size packages of chicken, fish, and steak.

2. Divide your meats and other proteins into individual servings, then place each serving into individual cooking pouches.

3. Don't forget to include your favorite seasonings before vacuum sealing the cooking pouch.

2 - Saving Time on Cooking

Cutting down on your cooking time has never been easier:

Cook, then freeze

- Season your food and place in the cooking pouches.

- Vacuum seal and place in the sous vide water oven to cook.

- Place the cooking pouches in an ice bath for thirty to forty-five minutes.

- Label the pouches with date and contents.

- Place in the freezer (use within a year).

- Take the pouch out of the freezer and thaw.

- Reheat for forty-five minutes for every inch of thickness.

- When reheating from frozen, reheat for thirty minutes more.

- Sear the reheated food and serve immediately with or without sauce.

Freeze, then cook

- Season your individual servings of fish, seafood, poultry, meat, or game.

- Place in the cooking pouches and vacuum seal.

- Write the date and contents on the label.

- Freeze the pouches with uncooked ingredients for no more than six weeks.

- Remove the pouches from the freezer and allow to thaw.

- Place in the sous vide water oven to cook at the target temperature.

- If cooking from frozen, cook for an additional thirty minutes.

- Serve sauced or seared.

Marinating

Marinate your foods with sous vide ease:

1. Place your fish/ meat/ poultry, vegetables, and other

ingredients in the cooking pouch. Add the marinade and then press with your hands (to remove air pockets) before sealing manually.

2. Place the cooking pouch in the freezer to allow the marinade to set.

3. Take the pouch out of the freezer and cut through the pouch (below the seal).

4. Vacuum seal the pouch and submerge in the sous vide water oven (preheated to target temperature). If cooking from frozen, allow to cook for an additional thirty minutes.

3 - Cooking Efficiently

Group similar food to save time:

Cooking vegetables

You can cook most vegetables in the temperature range of 183 degrees Fahrenheit to 185 degrees Fahrenheit. The food will generally become tender within forty-five minutes to one hour in the sous vide water oven.

To save time, you can submerge several cooking pouches containing different types of vegetables in the sous vide water oven all at once. You can then consume the cooked vegetables for several days. This trick may have you spending some hands-on veggie prepping time.

It does allow you to literally just leave them to cook on their own. While your sous vide water oven is cooking all the vegetables you need for the next three days, you can work on your exercise routine, play with your baby, or watch your favorite TV reruns.

Cooking meats

You can cook meats (beef, duck, lamb, ostrich, bison, and other red meats – placed inside different cooking pouches) at the same time and at the same sous vide water oven temperature of 134 degrees Fahrenheit (for that perfectly medium-rare doneness). Just keep in mind that the length of cooking time will vary, depending on the toughness as well as the thickness of the meat cut.

If you would rather have your meat cooked medium or well-done, simply set your sous vide water oven to 140 degrees or 150 degrees Fahrenheit. Any which way, you can rest assured that your meat will be cooked evenly from the center to the edges.

After seasoning your meats, portion them according to your needs and then place inside their cooking pouches. Vacuum seal before cooking all at once in the sous vide water oven at their target temperature.

Once cooked, remove the pouches from the sous vide water oven and place in an ice bath. Dry off the pouches before labeling with their respective dates and contents, then place in the refrigerator to chill for up to two days, or place in the freezer to keep for up to one year.

Cooking tougher meat cuts

Tougher meat cuts include spare ribs, roasts, and grass-fed

beef. Simply tenderize overnight by cooking for 8 to 10 hours or more.

Cooking poultry

You can cook chicken meat (or turkey) along with pork at the temperature range of 140 degrees Fahrenheit to 146 degrees Fahrenheit for two hours to two hours and thirty minutes. Submerge up to 12 chicken breasts, or 8 turkey breasts, or 6 pork tenderloins, or 16 pork chops, or any combination of these meats.

As soon as they are cooked, remove from the sous vide water oven and their cooking pouches, then submerge in an ice bath. Dry off and label before refrigerating for up to two days or freezing up to one year.

Reheating previously cooked food

While your fish is cooking in the sous vide water oven, you can add in pouches containing cooked veggies to reheat them. A ½-inch fish fillet's delicate flesh only requires 20 to 40 minutes of cooking, so you can drop and reheat one to two pouches of cooked veggies in the sous vide water oven as the fish cooks.

Doing it this way allows you to have delicious, nutritious, and effortless dinner ready within just 30 to 40 minutes.

Multitask cooking

As long as there is enough space in the sous vide water oven, you can cook pork spare ribs for thirty hours at 176 degrees along with chicken, turkey, or duck leg quarters (which also cook at the same target temperature).

4 - Succulent Sous Vide Fish for Dinner Recipes

Dill Caper and Artichoke Salmon

Ingredients:

Salmon:

- Kosher salt (1/2 cup)

- Dill, fresh, chopped (1 teaspoon)

- Liquid smoke, Applewood (1 tablespoon)

- Salmon steaks, boned removed, 2" (4 pieces)

- Brown sugar (1/2 cup)

- Pepper, freshly ground (1/2 teaspoon)

- Olive oil, extra virgin (2 tablespoons)

Artichokes:

- Lemon juice, freshly squeezed (1/2 tablespoon)

- Artichokes, trimmed, w/choke removed (4 pieces)

- Salt (1/4 teaspoon)

- Pepper, freshly ground (1/4 teaspoon)

Sauce:

- Butter, melted (4 ounces)

- Dill, fresh, chopped (1 tablespoon)

- Dijon mustard (1/2 teaspoon)

- Egg yolks (3 pieces)

- Capers, chopped (1 tablespoon)

- Salt (1/2 teaspoon + ¼ teaspoon)

- Lemon juice, freshly squeezed (1 tablespoon + ½ tablespoon)

Directions:

1. Place the pepper, sugar, and dill in a medium bowl. Add the salt and liquid smoke. Stir to combine into a paste. Rub all surfaces of the salmon steaks with the paste, making sure they are evenly covered. Place the salmon steaks on a large plate, then wrap with cling film before placing in the refrigerator for one hour.

2. Rinse the steaks thoroughly until all traces of the paste are gone. Use paper towels to pat dry afterwards. Working in batches, place the steaks inside cooking pouches. Vacuum seal the pouches before placing in the refrigerator until cooking time.

3. Fill the sous vide water oven and then preheat to 185 degrees.

4. Meanwhile, trim and peel the artichoke stems before rubbing with lemon juice. Place in a cooking pouch, vacuum seal, and submerge in the sous vide water oven. Cook for about one hour and fifteen minutes or until tenderly cooked. Transfer the pouch containing the artichokes onto a plate before lowering the sous vide water oven's temperature to 149 degrees.

5. Fill a cooking pouch with the ingredients for the sauce. Vacuum seal before submerging in the sous vide water oven to cook for forty-five minutes. Once done, transfer to a blender filled with capers and dill. Process until well-emulsified and thick, pour into a cooking pouch, and vacuum seal. Place in the sous vide water oven again to keep warm (do the same to

the cooked artichokes).

6. Lower the sous vide water oven temperature further to 134 degrees. Drop the pouch containing the chilled salmon steaks and allow to cook for one hour along with the artichokes and sauce.

7. In the meantime, heat a well-greased grill until extremely hot.

8. Once the salmon steaks are done. Then remove from the water oven and set on a tray. Do the same with the artichokes.

9. Brush a bit of olive oil on all sides of the salmon steaks and artichokes, then sprinkle pepper and salt on the artichokes alone. Place the salmon steaks on the grill and cook for thirty seconds on each side or until seared and golden; repeat with the artichokes. Once done, transfer onto a serving platter (warmed), making sure the artichokes surround the salmon.

10. Take the sauce out of the sous vide water oven and pour on top of the salmon steaks and artichokes. Serve right away.

Easy and Delicious Salmon

Ingredients:

- Kosher salt (1 ½ teaspoons)

- Butter, unsalted, sliced into 4 portions (28 grams)

- King salmon, skinless, boneless, 6 ounces (4 pieces)

- Lemon slices, fresh (4 pieces)

Directions:

1. Fill the sous vide water oven before preheating to 126 degrees.

2. Meanwhile, sprinkle salt on the salmon pieces before topping each with a slice of lemon and a portion of butter.

3. Transfer 2 salmon portions into a cooking pouch. Vacuum seal the two pouches before submerging in the sous vide water oven. Cook for twenty minutes.

4. Meanwhile, heat a skillet before adding a little oil.

5. Once the salmon is done, remove from the sous vide

water and transfer onto the hot, greased skillet. Cook for one to two minutes or until the salmon pieces are caramelized on the surface.

6. Serve and enjoy.

Yummy Cranberry Salmon

Ingredients:

- Cilantro, fresh, chopped (a handful)

- Salmon fillets, boneless, skinless, 5 ounces (2 pieces)

- Marinade:

- Barbecue sauce (2 tablespoons)

- Cranberry juice (1 tablespoon)

- Salt (1/8 teaspoon)

- Cranberry sauce (2 tablespoons)

- Olive oil, extra virgin (1 tablespoon)

- Lime juice, freshly squeezed (1 teaspoon)

Directions:

1. Place all the ingredients for the marinade in a medium bowl. Stir to combine. Set aside 1½ tablespoons of the mixture for using later in a separate step.

2. Place the salmon fillets in the marinade and coat with the mixture on all sides. Cover the bowl before placing in the refrigerator for one to two hours.

3. Meanwhile, fill the sous vide water oven before preheating to 140 degrees.

4. Take the marinated salmon fillets out of the refrigerator and transfer into a cooking pouch. Vacuum seal, place in the sous vide water oven and cook for twenty-five to thirty minutes.

5. Set the broiler on high to preheat.

6. Once the salmon fillets are done. Then transfer to a pan (broiler-safe). Coat with the marinade you set aside earlier before placing in the broiler. Cook for one to two minutes or until heated through.

7. Top with chopped cilantro and serve immediately. Enjoy.

Chili Maple and Lemon Salmon

Ingredients:

- Sea salt, spiced (1 ½ tablespoons)

- Parsley, curly, freshly chopped (4 tablespoons)

- Maple syrup (4 ounces)

- Leeks, chopped (1 2/3 cups)

- Lemon zest, finely grated (1 tablespoon)

- Salmon fillet, fresh, scaled, 2 ½-oz. (4 pieces)

- Castor sugar (1 ½ tablespoons)

- Double cream (3 tablespoons + 1 teaspoon)

- Red chili, small (1 piece)

- Lemons, halved, caramelized (2 pieces)

Directions:

1. Mix the sugar and salt together before sprinkling on
   the fish fillets. Place the seasoned fillets in a large
   bowl, cover, and refrigerate for two hours.

2. Meanwhile, fill the sous vide water oven before pre-heating to 115 degrees.

3. Take the chilled fish fillets out of the refrigerator and lightly rinse before patting dry with paper towels and placing inside cooking pouches. After vacuum sealing the pouches, submerge in the preheated sous vide water oven. Allow the fish fillets to cook for forty-five minutes.

4. In the meantime, heat a water-filled pan on high. Allow the water to boil before adding the chopped leeks and salt. Boil for another two to three minutes, then drain and rinse with cold water. Drain again before squeezing the leeks until thoroughly dry. Place in a small bowl and set aside.

5. Heat another pan on medium. Add the cream and allow to boil to slightly thicken it. Stir in the leeks and cook for one to two minutes or until warmed through. Stir in the black pepper and salt. Then reduce heat to low to keep the mixture warm.

6. Heat another saucepan (small) on medium after pouring in the maple syrup. Once the syrup is cara-

melized, cover the pan and set aside to keep warm.

7. Slice the chili into lengthwise halves before removing the stems and deseeding. Mince the flesh and stir into the maple syrup. Stir in the lemon zest, black pepper, and chopped parsley as well.

8. After taking the cooked salmon out of the sous vide water bath, pat dry with paper towels and brush with the maple syrup mixture.

9. Meanwhile, pour the leek mixture onto a platter. Add the salmon on top.

10. Serve drizzled with more maple syrup mixture and enjoy.

Italian Style Poached Cod

Ingredients:

Cod:

- Olive oil, extra virgin (3 tablespoons)

- Lemon zest (1/2 tablespoon)

- Cod fillets, skinless, 6-oz. (2 pieces)

- Parsley sprigs, fresh (2 pieces)

- Peppers & olives:

- Red peppers, roasted, chopped (1/3 cup)

- Black olives, sliced (1/3 cup)

- Salt, kosher (1/4 teaspoon)

- Pepper, freshly cracked (1/4 teaspoon)

- Onion, small, peeled, diced (1 piece)

- Rosemary, fresh, chopped finely (1 teaspoon)

- Red pepper flakes (a pinch)

Salsa:

- Garlic clove, peeled, crushed (1 piece)

- Balsamic vinegar (1 teaspoon)

- Salt, kosher (1/4 teaspoon)

- Pepper, freshly cracked (1/4 teaspoon)

- Plum tomatoes, sliced (1 ¼ cups)

- Olive oil, extra virgin (1 teaspoon)

- Paprika, smoked (1/4 teaspoon)

Directions:

1. Fill the sous vide water oven before preheating to 181 degrees.

2. Fill a cooking pouch (small) with the tomatoes. Add the olive oil and garlic, then vacuum seal and place in the sous vide water oven. Cook for forty-five minutes before transferring into the blender. Add the smoked paprika and vinegar, then process until well-blended and smooth. Season with pepper and salt before setting aside.

3. Lower the sous vide water oven's temperature to 132 degrees.

4. Heat a skillet on medium-high before adding olive oil. Stir in the diced onions and cook for three minutes or until translucent and fragrant. Add the red pepper, olives, and rosemary; stir to combine

with the onions. Reduce heat to medium and cook for an additional four to six minutes before sprinkling salt and pepper into the mixture. Remove from heat and set aside.

5. Place the fish inside a cooking pouch (large). Add the salt, pepper, and olive oil before vacuum sealing the pouch. Submerge into the sous vide water oven to cook for twenty minutes.

6. Meanwhile, pour the tomato mixture onto a plate. Once the fish is cooked, place on top of the tomato mixture. Pour the onions and olives over the fish before garnishing with fresh parsley.

7. Serve sprinkled with lemon zest.

5 - Evenly Tender Sous Vide Poultry for Dinner Recipes

Paleo Friendly Crispy Chicken

Ingredients:

- Butter, unsalted (6 tablespoons)

- Black pepper, freshly ground (1/2 teaspoon)

- Garlic powder (1/4 teaspoon)

- Thyme, dried (1/4 teaspoon)

- Kosher salt (1/4 teaspoon)

- Lard (2 tablespoons)

- Chicken thighs, boneless, skin-on (6 pieces)

Directions:

1. Fill the sous vide water oven before preheating to 150 degrees.

2. Pat the chicken thighs with paper towels to dry after flattening them. Season with pepper, salt, dried thyme, and garlic powder on the skinless side.

3. Rub butter (1 tablespoon) on each chicken thigh before placing inside the cooking pouch. Vacuum seal before submerging in the preheated sous vide water oven. Allow the chicken thighs to cook for one hour and thirty minutes.

4. Meanwhile, heat a skillet on medium before adding lard. Once the lard is smoking, add the cooked chicken thighs. With their skin sides down, cook for about three to five minutes or until the skins are crisp. Once done, allow the chicken thighs to drain on a wire rack after sprinkling the crisped skins with a little fleur de sel.

5. Place the chicken thighs alongside your favorite vegetables.

6. Serve and enjoy.

Extra Special Turkey

Ingredients:

- Water, filtered (2 quarts)

- Black peppercorns, whole (1 tablespoon)

- Butter (6 tablespoons)

- Turkey, whole, 10-pound (1 piece)

- Kosher salt (11 tablespoons)

- Poultry seasoning (1 tablespoon)

- Sage sprigs, fresh (3 pieces)

Directions:

1. Remove the breasts (with skin on) and leg quarters from the turkey and place in a large bowl; set aside. Reserve the carcass for making turkey stock later.

2. Meanwhile, fill a large pot with water. Add salt, poultry seasoning, and peppercorns; stir to combine.

3. Add the turkey pieces in the pot filled with herbed brine. Cover and place in the refrigerator to brine overnight.

4. Fill the sous vide water oven before preheating to 146 degrees.

5. Meanwhile, pat dry the turkey pieces with paper towels after rinsing well. Place each turkey piece in an in-

dividual cooking pouch. To each pouch, add 1 sage sprig and 2 tablespoons of butter before vacuum sealing.

6. Place the turkey leg quarters in the refrigerator while you cook the turkey breasts first. Submerge the breast pouches in the sous vide water oven; cook for four to six hours. Once done, transfer the breast pouches into an ice bath for a minimum of one hour (alternatively, you can place them in the refrigerator for no more than two days prior to finishing).

7. Raise the sous vide water oven's temperature to 176 degrees. Add the cooking pouches containing the leg quarters and cook for eight to twelve hours. Once done, transfer into an ice bath or refrigerate for one to two days prior to finishing.

8. Fill the sous vide water oven and then preheat to 146 degrees. Drop the breast pouches as well as leg quarter pouches for a minimum of one hour. Once the turkey pieces are reheated, remove from their pouches and pat dry using paper towels. Brush all sides with herbed butter (melted) and set aside.

9. Heat the broiler on high. Cook the turkey pieces for a few minutes or until the skins are seared and golden brown.

10. Serve and enjoy.

Arborio and Cremini Turkey

Ingredients:

- Olive oil, extra virgin (1 teaspoon)

- Garlic, minced, roasted (2 tablespoons)

- Salt, kosher (1/4 teaspoon)

- Pepper, freshly cracked (1/4 teaspoon)

- Cremini mushrooms, cleaned, sliced (10 pieces)

- Rosemary leaves, fresh, minced (1 tablespoon)

- Arborio rice (1 cup)

- Yellow onion, small, peeled, diced (1 piece)

- Turkey, cooked, diced (8 ounces)

- Turkey broth, reduced sodium (3 cups)

- Romano cheese, grated (1/3 cup)

Directions:

1. Fill the sous vide water oven before preheating to 183 degrees.

2. Heat a large skillet over medium. Then add the olive oil. Once heated through, stir in onions and mushrooms. Cook for four to five minutes or until tender and fragrant.

3. Transfer the sautéed onions and mushrooms into a cooking pouch (gallon size). Add all the other ingredients (save for the cheese) for this recipe before vacuum sealing the pouch.

4. Place the sealed pouch in the preheated sous vide water oven. Allow the mixture in the pouch to cook for forty-five minutes. Once done, transfer the pouch contents to a serving bowl (pre-warmed).

5. Use a fork to fluff the cooked rice before stirring in the cheese.

6. Serve right away.

Onion Chicken

Ingredients:

- Mustard oil (3 tablespoons + 1 teaspoon)

- Yogurt, natural, salted (4 ounces)

- Chicken breasts, boneless (2 pounds)

- Cilantro, fresh (a handful)

- Mint leaves, fresh (a handful)

Marinade:

- Ground coriander, powdered (1 tablespoon)

- Fenugreek, dry (1 teaspoon)

- Cilantro, fresh, chopped, divided (1 handful)

- Ginger garlic paste (2 tablespoons)

- Greek yogurt, low-fat, plain (3 tablespoons)

- Garam masala (2 tablespoons)

- Cayenne pepper, ground (1 teaspoon)

- Lemon juice, freshly squeezed (1 tablespoon)

- Food coloring, bright orange (1/4 teaspoon)

- Salt, kosher (1/4 teaspoon)

Onions:

- Fenugreek, dry (1 teaspoon)

- Red onions, large, peeled, sliced thinly (2 pieces)

- Balsamic vinegar (2 tablespoons)

- Olive oil, extra virgin (1 tablespoon)

- Salt, kosher (1/4 teaspoon)

- Brown sugar (1 tablespoon)

Directions:

1. Pat dry the chicken breasts after rinsing, then set aside.

2. Place the ingredients (set aside ½ of the fresh cori-ander for using later) for the marinade in a large bowl. Add the chicken breasts, turning to ensure all

sides are evenly coated with the marinade. Cover and place in the refrigerator to marinate for two hours.

3. Meanwhile, fill the sous vide water oven and preheat to 160 degrees.

4. Drain off all traces of marinade before placing the chicken breasts inside a cooking pouch. Vacuum seal and then place in the preheated sous vide water oven. Cook for two to three hours.

5. Meanwhile, heat a frying pan (nonstick) on medium-low. Add the olive oil and then stir in the onions. Add the salt and fenugreek, then sauté for about fifteen to twenty minutes or until onions are tender and cara-melized. Stir in the balsamic vinegar as well as brown sugar, making sure the onions are well-coated. Once done, remove from heat and set aside.

6. Take the cooked chicken breasts out of the cooking pouch and drain. Pat dry with paper towels and place on a plate.

7. Heat a skillet (nonstick) on medium-high before adding the mustard oil. Once heated through, add the

chicken pieces and cook on each side for one to two minutes or until golden brown and nicely seared.

8. Transfer the chicken pieces onto a platter, alongside the caramelized onions. Top with fresh mint leaves and the reserved fresh coriander.

9. Serve and enjoy.

Easy Herbed Turkey with Cranberry Sauce

Ingredients:

- Salt, kosher (4 tablespoons)

- Butter, unsalted, divided (3 tablespoons)

- Black pepper, freshly ground (1/4 teaspoon)

- Olive oil, extra virgin (1 tablespoon)

- Water (2 cups)

- Black peppercorns (10 pieces)

- Sage leaves, fresh (4 pieces)

- Garlic cloves, roasted, minced finely (2 pieces)

- Cranberry sauce:

- Sugar, granulated (1 cup)

- Cranberries, fresh (12 ounces)

- Orange zest, freshly grated (1 tablespoon)

Directions:

1. Fill the sous vide water oven before preheating to 183 degrees.

2. Fill a cooking pouch with all the ingredients for the cranberry sauce. Vacuum seal before submerging in the preheated sous vide water oven to cook for one hour. Once the mixture is done, take the pouch out of the sous vide water oven and smash gently with your hands to make the cranberry sauce chunky. Quickly submerge the cranberry sauce pouch into an ice bath. After twenty minutes, place in the refrigerator for two to three days.

3. Fill a large cooking pouch (gallon size) with water and salt. Once the salt is dissolved, add the turkey

breast and peppercorns. Vacuum seal the pouch and place in the refrigerator for four hours to allow the turkey to brine.

4. Meanwhile, fill the sous vide water oven and preheat to 146 degrees.

5. Rinse the brined turkey before patting dry with paper towels. Sprinkle black pepper on all sides of the turkey and place inside a cooking pouch. Add butter (2 tablespoons), sage leaves, and garlic before vacuum sealing and submerging in the sous vide water oven. Allow the turkey to cook for three to four hours. Once done, pour the pouch juices into a small bowl and set aside for making gravy/sauce later. Pat dry the chicken pieces and set aside on a large plate.

6. Heat the broiler on high. Meanwhile, brush all surfaces of the cooked turkey with the remaining butter (melted). Broil the turkey for five minutes or until the skin is nicely browned and crisp. Once done, transfer onto a serving platter (warmed).

7. Serve drenched in cranberry sauce. Enjoy.

6 - Mouthwatering Sous Vide Beef for Dinner Recipes

Pesto and Asparagus Beef

Ingredients:

- Basil leaves, fresh (1 cup)

- Salt, kosher, divided (1 tablespoon)

- Lemon zest, freshly grated (1/2 tablespoon)

- Lemon juice, freshly squeezed (1/2 tablespoon)

- Olive oil, extra virgin (1/4 cup)

- Asparagus spears (20 pieces)

- Beef tenderloin, grass-fed, 6-oz. (4 pieces)

- Black pepper, freshly cracked (1/2 teaspoon)

- Garlic cloves, large, fresh, peeled (5 pieces)

- Parmesan cheese, grated (2 tablespoons)

Directions:

1. Fill the sous vide water oven before preheating to 134

degrees.

2. Meanwhile, sprinkle pepper and salt on the meat before placing inside cooking pouches (2 meat portions
   per pouch). Vacuum seal and then place in the sous
   vide water oven; allow the meat to cook for two
   hours.

3. Fill a pot with water and heat on high until boiling.
   Drop the basil leaves; after thirty seconds, remove
   and transfer immediately into an ice bath. Wring dry
   before chopping roughly and set aside in a blender.
   Do the same to the garlic.

4. In the blender, add the olive oil, salt (1 teaspoon), and
   Parmesan cheese. Process until well-combined and
   smooth before adding the lemon juice.

5. Meanwhile, fill a cooking pouch with the asparagus,
   making sure the asparagus pieces form a single layer.
   Add a little salt and 1/3 of the basil mixture. Vacuum
   seal and then drop into the sous vide water oven. Allow the asparagus to cook along with the meat for fifteen minutes. Once done, remove the steak and asparagus from the cooking pouches, and set aside on a

large plate.

6. Heat a grill pan on high before adding a little oil. Once heated through, add the steaks to sear on each side for about thirty to forty-five seconds. Transfer on a platter alongside the asparagus.

7. Serve topped with the remaining basil mixture (2/3 portion) and serve immediately.

Wagyu Fillets with Green Beans

Ingredients:

- Vegetable oil, high smoke point (1 tablespoon)

- Rosemary sprigs, fresh, divided (2 pieces)

- Beef tenderloin filets, Wagyu, 2-inches thick (2 pieces)

- Green beans, cooked (1 ½ cups)

- Butter, unsalted (2 tablespoons)

- Salt, kosher (1/4 teaspoon)

- Pepper, freshly cracked (1/4 teaspoon)

Directions:

1. Fill the sous vide water oven before preheating to 130 degrees. Meanwhile, fill a small cooking pouch with the cooked green beans.

2. Sprinkle pepper and salt on the fillets before placing them inside a cooking pouch (quart-size). After adding a rosemary sprig, vacuum seal the pouch and place in the sous vide water oven. Cook for two hours and thirty minutes to four hours.

3. Thirty minutes before the fillets' cooking time ends, add the pouch containing the green beans to the sous vide water oven.

4. Once done, take the fillets and green beans out of the sous vide water oven and transfer onto large plates. Use paper towels to pat dry the fillets. Set aside.

5. Heat a skillet on high before adding the vegetable oil. Once heated through, add the cooked fillets and sear for one minute on each side. Flip the fillets before adding in the butter as well as remaining rosemary sprig. Cook the fillets in the butter until basted and

crusted on all sides.

6. Serve the fillets alongside green beans and enjoy.

Western Style Burger

Ingredients:

Burger:

- Gorgonzola picante (1 ounce)

- Ground chuck, Angus (10 ounces)

- Frying oil, high smoke point (2 cups)

- Barbecue sauce (2 ounces)

- Butter (1 tablespoon)

- Pork roast (1/2 pound)

- Salt, kosher (1/4 teaspoon)

- Pepper, freshly cracked (1/4 teaspoon)

- Jalapeno peppers, fresh (2 pieces)

- Bread, focaccia (2 pieces)

Onion rings:

- Paprika, Spanish (1/2 tablespoon)

- Cornstarch (1/2 cup)

- Pale ale (15 ounces)

- Cayenne pepper (1/2 teaspoon)

- Baking soda (2 teaspoons)

- Flour, all purpose, bleached (2 cups)

- Black pepper, freshly ground (1 teaspoon)

- Salt, kosher (2 ½ tablespoons)

- Baking powder (2 tablespoons)

- Yellow onion, large, peeled, sliced into quarter-inch slices (1 piece)

Directions:

1. Fill the sous vide water oven before preheating to 140 degrees.

2. Fill a small cooking pouch (quart size) with the pork.

Pour in the barbecue sauce before vacuum sealing the pouch. Drop in the sous vide water oven and allow the pork t cook for one to two days.

3. Sprinkle pepper and salt on the chuck burger, then mold into 2 patties. Place the patties inside a cooking pouch and freeze, unsealed, for two to three hours or until firm.

4. Meanwhile, decrease the water bath temperature to 130 degrees by adding ice cubes or iced water.

5. Take the patties out of the freezer. After vacuum sealing the pouch, place it in the sous vide water oven. Along with the pork, cook the patties for a minimum of one hour.

6. Heat a large skillet on medium-high before adding the oil (2 inches deep). In the meantime, sprinkle the onion slices with pepper and salt before dusting liberally with a small portion of the flour.

7. Place the rest of the flour in a large bowl. Add all the remaining ingredients to the batter. Stir continuously until well-combined and no lumps remain in the pan-

cake batter.

8. Once the oil temperature in the skillet reaches 350 degrees, add the onion slices (after being dipped into the prepared batter) and cook for about two to four minutes or until golden brown and crisp.

9. Remove the cooked onion slices. Add the fresh jalapeno and quickly toss in the oil. Once done (the skin is blistered), transfer onto a small dish.

10. As soon as the burgers are almost done, heat a broiler on high. Add the burgers and briefly cook until nicely seared and a bit charred on the surface.

11. Slice the focaccia into halves, then spread the cut sides with butter. Add to the broiler and sear, butter side down, alongside the burgers.

12. Place the unbuttered focaccia pieces on a platter. Brush a bit of barbecue sauce on the surface before topping with the patties and additional sauce, as well as pork and crumbled gorgonzola. Finish off each burger by adding an onion ring as well as a fried jalapeno and the buttered focaccia half.

13. Serve and enjoy.

Divine Smoked Beef

Ingredients:

- Beef brisket, trimmed (6 pounds)

- Meat rub (1/2 cup) – see below

Meat rub:

- Brown sugar (1 tablespoon)

- Salt, coarse (2 tablespoons)

- Onion powder (1 teaspoon)

- Paprika (3 tablespoons)

- Black pepper, freshly ground (1 tablespoon)

- Garlic powder (1 teaspoon)

- Cumin, ground (1 teaspoon)

Directions:

1. After filling the sous vide water oven with water, set

to 134 degrees to preheat.

2. Follow manufacturer's directions in setting up your device with hickory chips/ cakes/ pellets. For five minutes, use smoke produced by a smoking gun following food preparation.

3. Meanwhile, combine all ingredients for the meat rub in a medium bowl. Use this mixture to coat the brisket generously on all sides.

4. Place the seasoned brisket inside the cooking pouch. Vacuum seal before dropping the pouch inside the sous vide water oven. Allow the brisket to cook for forty-eight hours.

5. Once the brisket is done, remove the cooking pouch from the sous vide water oven and take out the brisket. Place in a closed container and smoke for thirty seconds. Allow the meat to soak up the smoke for five minutes.

6. Meanwhile, heat a skillet on high. Add the smoked brisket and cook for thirty to forty-five seconds or until the surface is crisp, seared, and caramelized.

7. After slicing, serve immediately and enjoy.

Smashing Ribs with Mashers

Ingredients:

Ribs:

- Salt, kosher (1/4 teaspoon)

- Pepper, freshly cracked (1/4 teaspoon)

- Celery stalk, trimmed, diced (1 piece)

- Tomato paste (2 tablespoons)

- Olive oil, extra virgin (1 tablespoon)

- Garlic cloves, peeled, minced (2 pieces)

- Red wine (4 ounces)

- Short ribs, 3-inches (4 pieces)

- Onion, peeled, diced (1/2 piece)

- Carrot, peeled, diced (1 piece)

- Thyme sprig (1 piece)

- Oil – to be used in searing

Mashers:

- Salt, kosher (1/4 teaspoon)

- Pepper, freshly cracked (1/4 teaspoon)

- Cream (2 ounces)

- Cheddar cheese (2 ounces)

- Red potatoes, creamer (1 pound)

- Butter (2 ounces)

- Chives, fresh, minced (1 tablespoon)

Directions:

1. Fill the sous vide water oven with water before setting to 185 degrees to preheat.

2. Rub pepper and salt on the short ribs, making sure all sides are seasoned well.

3. Heat a skillet (nonstick) on medium-high before adding the oil. Once heated through, add the

seasoned short ribs and cook until all sides are seared and browned. Once the ribs are done, transfer to a plate and cover to keep warm.

4. Wipe the pan before adding in olive oil (1 tablespoon). Stir in the vegetables and sauté until browned. Stir in the tomato paste as well and cook for one minute before pouring in the wine. Lower heat to medium and allow mixture to simmer until reduced. Transfer the mixture to a large bowl and place in the refrigerator for thirty minutes.

5. Pour the vegetable mixture into a cooking pouch. Add the ribs on top, making sure they form a single layer. Vacuum seal the pouch and place inside the sous vide water oven to cook for twelve hours.

6. Meanwhile, place the potatoes at the bottom of a cooking pouch. Sprinkle in the seasoning before vacuum sealing and dropping into the sous vide water oven. Allow the potatoes to cook for one hour before taking out of the water oven. Roughly press on the cooked potatoes (through the pouch) until mashed before slipping in the remaining ingredients. Mix well

and divide the potato mixture among 4 individual plates.

7. Take the cooked ribs out of the sous vide water oven. Place one rib on top of each masher-filled plate.

8. Meanwhile, pour the rib juices (from the pouch in which you cooked the ribs) into a pan. Heat on medium and cook until reduced. Drizzle the reduced liquid on top of the ribs.

9. Serve and enjoy.

7 - Scrumptious Sous Vide Pork for Dinner Recipes

Barbecue Pork Ribs

Ingredients:

- Olive oil, extra virgin – for cooking

- Ribs, country style, meaty (8 pieces)

- Barbecue sauce – see below

- Barbecue sauce:

- Salad oil (1 cup)

- Garlic, granulated (3 tablespoons)

- Pepper, white (2 tablespoons)

- Lemon juice (4 tablespoons)

- Salt, kosher (3 tablespoons)

- Ketchup (114 ounces)

- Cumin, ground (2 tablespoons)

- Oregano, dry (2 teaspoons)

- Molasses (1 cup)

- Black pepper, freshly ground (1 tablespoon)

- Onions, medium, peeled, minced (4 pieces)

- Brown sugar (2 ½ pounds)

- Cider vinegar (1 quart)

- Mustard, dry (4 tablespoons)

- Chile powder (1/3 cup)

- Cayenne pepper (1 tablespoon)

- Tabasco sauce (3 ounces)

- Honey (1 cup)

- Thyme, dry (1 tablespoon)

Meat rub:

- Sugar, granulated (2 tablespoons)

- Chile powder (2 tablespoons)

- Cayenne pepper (2 teaspoons)

- Cumin (2 tablespoons)

- Black pepper, freshly ground (1 tablespoon)

- Salt, kosher (1/4 cup)

- Paprika (2 tablespoons)

- Garlic powder (2 tablespoons)

- Mustard powder (1 tablespoon)

Directions:

1. Heat a soup pot (large) on medium before adding the salad oil. Once heated through, stir in the onions as well as brown sugar (1 tablespoon). Cook for five minutes or until the onions are caramelized.

2. Add the rest of the barbecue ingredients. Then stir well until the mixture is evenly combined. Turn heat down to low and allow the mixture to simmer for about an hour. Once done, pour the barbecue sauce into an airtight jar and place in the refrigerator.

3. Meanwhile, fill the sous vide water oven before pre-heating to 160 degrees.

4. Fill a small mixing bowl with the ingredients for the rib rub, Stir to combine and set aside.

5. Drizzle olive oil on the ribs before liberally brushing all sides with the prepared rib rub. Place the ribs inside large cooking pouches, making sure they form a single layer and then vacuum seal.

6. Drop the cooking pouches into the sous vide water oven. Allow the ribs to cook for eighteen to twenty-four hours.

7. Once the ribs are done, remove from the cooking pouches and set on a platter. Smother with the barbecue sauce and serve immediately.

Veggies and Pork with Blueberry Sauce and Sweet Potato Puree

Ingredients:

- Pork belly slab, 8-oz. (1 piece)

- Marinade:

- Cumin (1 teaspoon)

- Black pepper, freshly cracked (1 teaspoon)

- Fennel seeds (1 teaspoon)

- Cayenne pepper (1 tablespoon)

- Olive oil, extra virgin (1/4 cup)

- Salt, kosher (2 teaspoons)

- Cinnamon (1 tablespoon)

- Cloves, whole (3 pieces)

- Soy sauce, reduced sodium (1/2 cup)

Sweet potato puree:

- Butter, unsalted (2 tablespoons)

- Sweet potato, white, peeled, diced (1 piece)

- Cream (1/4 cup)

- Blueberry sauce:

- Sugar (1/4 cup)

- Vegetable stock (1/4 cup)

- Butter, unsalted (1 tablespoon)

- Blueberries, fresh/ frozen (1/2 cup)

- Soy sauce, low sodium (1 splash)

- Sesame chili oil (1/2 teaspoon)

Veggies:

- Mushrooms, wood ear (8 pieces)

- Mushrooms, nameko (4 ounces)

- Peppers, shishito (8 pieces)

- Vegetable stock (1 tablespoon)

- Butter, unsalted (1 tablespoon)

Directions:

1. Place the pork belly in a large bowl. Season with a mixture of pepper, cayenne, salt, cumin, and cinnamon. Add the fennel seeds, cloves, olive oil, and soy sauce, then toss until well-combined. Cover and place in the refrigerator to marinate overnight.

2. Fill the sous vide water oven before preheating to 155 degrees.

3. Remove the marinated pork belly from the refrigerator. Drain the marinade and then pat the meat with paper towels to dry. Transfer into a cooking pouch, vacuum seal, and drop into the sous vide water oven. Allow the pork belly to cook for four hours.

4. Meanwhile, heat a large pot on medium-high. Add salt (1 teaspoon) and bring water to a boil. Once boiling, add the potatoes; return to boiling and cook until tender.

5. Once the potatoes are done, strain and place in the food processor. Add salt, cream, and butter, then process until the potato mixture is well-combined. Return to the pot (after discarding the water) and heat on low to keep warm until served.

6. Heat a saucepot (1-quart) on medium-high before adding the sugar and blueberries. Once the sugar begins melting, gently mash the blueberries. Stir in the vegetable stock as well as sesame chili oil and soy sauce; cook for about two minutes or until heated

through.

7. Transfer the blueberry mixture into the food processor. Process until well-blended and then strain into the saucepot. Heat on medium and allow the blueberry mixture to cook until reduced to 1/2 and thickened. Once done, remove from heat and set aside.

8. Heat a saucepan on high before adding a little oil. Once heated through, stir in the shishito peppers as well as mushrooms. Cook for one minute before stirring in the vegetable stock (1 tablespoon). Allow the entire mixture to cook until reduced. Then stir in the butter (1 tablespoon). Once the butter has melted into the mixture, remove from heat and set aside.

9. Once the pork belly is done, remove from the sous vide water oven and cooking pouch, then transfer onto a plate. Set the pouch juices aside in a covered container.

10. Meanwhile, heat a frying pan on high before adding oil. Once the oil is heated through, add the pork belly and cook until the skin is seared. Gradually add the

reserved pouch juices and continue cooking until the pork belly is basted and its skin is crispy.

11. Serve and enjoy.

Brazilian Style Black Bean Stew

Ingredients:

- Onion, small, peeled, chopped (1 piece)

- Tomatoes, medium, trimmed, diced (3 pieces)

- Pork ribs, meaty, cooked, w/ meat pulled from bone (4 pieces)

- Sweet potato, medium, peeled, sliced (1 piece)

- Black beans, rinsed well (1 cup)

- Mango, peeled, seeded, cubed (1 piece)

- Bacon slices, thick, diced (4 pieces)

- Garlic clove, peeled, minced (1 piece)

- Red bell pepper, small, stemmed, seeded, diced (1 piece)

- Stock, vegetable/ stock (3 cups)

- Salt, kosher (1/4 teaspoon)

- Pepper, freshly cracked (1/4 teaspoon)

- Sausages, sweet, cooked, sliced (2 pieces)

Garnish:

- Arroz Braziliero, cooked (2 cups)

- Cilantro, fresh, chopped (a handful)

- Orange, fresh, sliced (1 piece)

Directions:

1. Fill the sous vide water oven before preheating to 195 degrees.

2. Meanwhile, heat a skillet on medium. Once hot, add the bacon and cook until browned and crisp.

3. Stir in the garlic and onions; cook for an additional two minutes or until fragrant and translucent. Turn off heat and allow the bacon mixture to slightly cool down.

4. Fill a large cooking pouch (1 gallon) with the bacon mixture as well as tomatoes, sweet potatoes, black beans, salt, pepper, red bell pepper, and vegetable stock. Vacuum seal before submerging into the pre-heated sous vide water oven and cook for three hours.

5. Meanwhile, fill another cooking pouch with the mangoes and cooked meats. Vacuum seal and drop into the sous vide water oven (after lowering its temperature to 158 degrees). Allow to warm along with the beans for half an hour.

6. Once done, transfer everything into a tureen (warmed). Stir to combine all cooked items. Serve topped with cilantro, orange, and Arroz Braziliero.

7. Enjoy.

Sage and Rosemary Pork Belly with Onions and Potatoes

Ingredients:

- Pork belly, rind on (1 pound)

- Olive oil, extra virgin (1 tablespoon)

- Sage, fresh, chopped roughly (1 teaspoon)

- Sea salt (1/4 teaspoon)

- Black pepper, freshly ground (1/4 teaspoon)

- Rosemary leaves, fresh (1 teaspoon)

Potatoes:

- White onion, medium, peeled, minced (1 piece)

- White wine, dry (1/2 cup)

- Sea salt (1/4 teaspoon)

- Pepper, freshly cracked (1/4 teaspoon)

- Olive oil, extra virgin (3 tablespoons)

- Potatoes, medium, peeled, chopped (3 pieces)

- Broth, beef, reduced sodium (2 cups)

Onions:

- Olive oil, extra virgin (4 tablespoons + 1 tablespoon)

- Water, filtered (2 ½ cups)

- Sea salt (1/4 teaspoon)

- Pepper, freshly cracked (1/4 teaspoon)

- Onions, cipollini, peeled (12 pieces)

- Vinegar, white wine (1/2 cup)

- Vinegar, balsamic (1 tablespoon)

Directions:

1. Heat a skillet on medium before adding the oil. Sauté for about five minutes or until a bit golden. Season with pepper and salt before pouring in the vinegar. Add the sugar as well. Then stir everything to combine. Allow the mixture to cook for five minutes or until all traces of vinegar are gone. Add water before covering and reducing heat to low. After five minutes, transfer the onions into a skillet greased with a little olive oil and heated on high. Add balsamic vinegar then cook until caramelized. Pour into a medium bowl and set aside.

2. Heat a medium gauge pot (heavy bottomed) on low before adding oil. Stir in the onion and cook for six to

eight minutes or until softened and fragrant. Stir in the potatoes and cook for another five minutes, making sure they are evenly coated. Pour in the white wine, stir, and allow to evaporate before pouring in the broth. Cook until the entire mixture is heated through and the potatoes are tender. Season with pepper and salt, then process into a puree with an immersion blender, food processor, or blender. Set aside in a large bowl.

3. Fill the sous vide water oven before preheating to 147 degrees.

4. Meanwhile, place the ingredients for the seasoning in a medium bowl. Stir to combine. Then rub the mixture all over the pork belly. Place the pork belly inside a cooking pouch, then vacuum seal and place in the preheated sous vide water oven to cook for eighteen to twenty-four hours.

5. Once the pork belly is done, take it out of the pouch and slice into 4 one-inch-thick portions. Set aside on a plate.

6. In the meantime, heat a heavy skillet (cast iron) on

high. Add olive oil and once heated through, add the pork belly with its rind side down. Cook until the rind is nicely seared, crunchy and golden.

7. Serve and enjoy.

Grilled Pork Ribs

Ingredients:

- Pork ribs, boneless (1 pound)

- Oregano, Mexican (1 tablespoon)

- Garlic cloves, peeled, chopped (2 pieces)

- Orange juice, freshly squeezed (1 cup)

- Onion, purple, peeled, sliced into rounds (1/2 piece)

- Achiote paste (2 ounces)

- Sazon seasoning, w/ salt, pepper & cumin (1 table-spoon)

- Vinegar, apple cider (1/2 cup)

- Olive oil, extra virgin (1/2 cup)

- Orange, sliced into rounds (1 piece)

Directions:

1. Fill the sous vide water oven before preheating to 149 degrees.

2. Pour the orange juice into a large bowl. Add the achiote paste, Sazon seasoning, and oregano, then whisk to combine into a smooth paste. Pour in the vinegar and whisk again to combine. Set aside.

3. Fill a large cooking pouch with the ribs. Pour in the prepared marinade as well as olive oil and garlic. Vacuum seal before submerging the pouch into the sous vide water oven. Allow the ribs to cook for twenty-four to forty-eight hours.

4. Heat a grill pan on high after generously oiling it. Once the ribs are tenderly done, transfer from the pouch and onto the grill pan to cook until both sides are seared.

5. Serve pork ribs with veggies on the side. Enjoy.

8 - Appetizing Sous Vide Lamb for Dinner Recipes

Lamb with Heirloom Tomatoes

Ingredients:

- Cherry tomatoes (1 pint)

- Salt, kosher, divided (1 tablespoon)

- Olive oil, extra virgin (1/4 cup)

- Rosemary sprigs, fresh (2 pieces)

- Chile flakes (1 teaspoon)

- Lamb rack, fresh (1 piece)

- Black pepper, freshly ground (1 teaspoon)

- Mint (1/2 bunch)

- Garlic cloves, peeled (2 pieces)

Directions:

1. Fill the sous vide water oven and then preheat to 136 degrees.

2. Meanwhile, sprinkle pepper and salt on the lamb, making sure all sides are evenly coated. Place inside a cooking pouch along with the rosemary sprigs, before vacuum sealing.

3. Drop the cooking pouch into the sous vide water oven. Allow the lamb to cook for two hours.

4. In the meantime, heat a pan on medium before adding olive oil. Add the garlic (thinly sliced), stir, and simmer for about three minutes. Once done, transfer into a cooking pouch along with the tomatoes, remaining salt, chile flakes, and mint. Vacuum seal and drop into the sous vide water oven as well to cook for one hour.

5. Once the lamb and tomato mixture are both done, remove from their pouches and transfer onto plates.

6. Heat a generously oiled grill pan on high before adding the lamb. Cook until all sides are seared, then transfer onto a platter. Set aside.

7. Meanwhile, drain the oil from the cooked tomatoes. After discarding the mint, place the tomatoes along-

side the lamb.

8. Serve and enjoy.

Lamb with Fig Syrup

Ingredients:

Lamb:

- Garlic cloves, peeled, minced (2 pieces)

- Cayenne, divided (1 teaspoon)

- Fennel pollen (2 tablespoons)

- Lamb racks, half ribs (2 pieces)

- Vegetable oil (1/4 cup)

- Rosemary, chopped finely (4 tablespoons)

- Black pepper, freshly ground (1 teaspoon)

- Salt, kosher, divided (2 ½ teaspoons)

Syrup:

- Fig preserves (1/2 cup)

- Vinegar, champagne (1/4 cup)

- Maple syrup, pure (1/4 cup)

Garnish:

- Walnuts, roasted, chopped finely (4 ounces)

- Goat cheese, young, crumbled (10 ounces)

- Parsley, Italian, chopped roughly (5 tablespoons)

Directions:

1. Fill the sous vide water oven before preheating to 134 degrees.

2. Place salt (2 teaspoons), garlic, pepper, cayenne (1/2 teaspoon), oil, fennel pollen, and rosemary in a medium bowl. Stir to combine.

3. Pat the lamb racks with paper towels to dry before rubbing the prepared spice mixture on all sides. Place inside a cooking pouch, then vacuum seal and submerge in the preheated sous vide water oven. Allow the lamb racks to cook for eighteen hours.

4. Meanwhile, fill a large saucepan (heavy bottomed)

with vinegar, salt (1/2 teaspoon), maple syrup, cayenne (1/2 teaspoon), and fig preserves. Stir to combine and then heat on medium. Allow the mixture to simmer before removing from heat and setting aside.

5. Once the lamb racks are done, remove from the sous vide water oven. Open the cooking pouch and slip the racks onto a large plate.

6. Heat a grill on high after generously greasing it with oil. Coat the lamb racks with fig syrup before cooking on the grill until nicely seared and browned.

7. Transfer the grilled lamb racks onto a platter. Coat again with fig syrup before slicing between the bones.

8. Transfer the ribs onto individual plates, making sure the ribs are evenly stacked. Top with chopped walnuts, crumbled goat cheese, and Italian parsley.

9. Serve and enjoy.

Pomegranate-Coffee Lamb

Ingredients:

- Brown sugar, packed (1/4 cup)

- Pepper, freshly cracked (1/4 teaspoon)

- Salt, kosher (1/4 teaspoon)

- Pomegranate juice (2 cups)

- Butter (1 tablespoon)

- Coffee, warm (1 cup)

- Balsamic vinegar (1/4 cup)

- Lamb racks, 1-oz. (2 pieces)

- Rosemary sprigs, fresh (2 pieces)

Directions:

- Place the brown sugar in a large bowl. Add the warm coffee and stir well. Once all the sugar granules are completely dissolved, add the pomegranate juice and balsamic vinegar. Stir again until well-combined, then reserve one cup of the mixture for using later (place in a small covered bowl and refrigerate).

- Place the 2 lamb racks in a large cooking pouch. Pour

in the remaining marinade and vacuum seal. Place in the refrigerator to marinate for four to twelve hours.

- Meanwhile, fill the sous vide water oven before pre-heating to 132 degrees.

- Drain the marinated lamb racks. Then pat dry with paper towels to remove any excess marinade. Season all sides of the racks with pepper and salt before placing into separate cooking pouches (gallon size). Include a fresh rosemary sprig in each cooking pouch before vacuum sealing, then drop into the sous vide water oven. Let the lamb racks cook for two hours.

- Meanwhile, take the reserved marinate out of the refrigerator. Pour into a skillet and heat on medium. Allow the marinade to boil before cooking for another five minutes or until reduced and thickened. Add the salt (1/8 teaspoon) and butter, whisk well until well-combined, and set aside.

- Set the broiler on high to preheat.

- Take the lamb pouches out if the sous vide water oven. Remove the racks from their pouches and transfer to a large pan (broiler safe). Cook under the broiler for four to five minutes or until all sides are seared and browned.

- Place the broiled lamb racks in the skillet where you cooked the sauce. Turn the racks to make sure all sides are evenly coated. Then slice each rack into single chops.

- Serve right away with additional sauce on the side.

- Enjoy.

Salsa Verde Lamb Croquettes

Ingredients:

- Olive oil, extra virgin – as needed in cooking

- Thyme sprigs, fresh (4 pieces)

- Eggs, beaten slightly w/ 1 tbsp. of water (2 pieces)

- Pepper, freshly cracked (1/4 teaspoon)

- Breadcrumbs, panko (1 cup)

- Veal demi-glace (1/4 cup)

- Flour, all-purpose (1/4 cup) – for dusting before breading

- Lamb shanks (2 pieces)

- Salt, kosher (1/4 teaspoon)

- Salsa verde – see below

Salsa verde:

- Parsley, fresh, chopped coarsely (1 cup)

- Lemon zest, freshly grated (1 tablespoon)

- Salt, kosher (1/4 teaspoon)

- Basil, fresh, chopped (2 tablespoons)

- Olive oil, extra virgin (2/3 cup)

- Garlic cloves, medium, unpeeled (6 pieces)

- Anchovy fillets, blotted w/ paper towels to remove oil (4 pieces)

- Tarragon, fresh, chopped (1 tablespoon)

- Egg yolks (3 pieces)

- Pepper, freshly ground (1/4 teaspoon)

Directions:

1. Fill a small saucepan with cold water (1/2 inch deep). Add the garlic and cover the pan before heating on high. Once boiling, discard the water and add fresh water (1/2 inch deep). Allow to boil again before removing the garlic and rinsing under cold water. Once the garlic is cool enough to work with, remove its skin and chop into bits.

2. Place the chopped garlic in the food processor. Add the lemon zest, anchovies, tarragon, parsley, egg yolks, and basil. Process while you gradually stream in the oil. Once the mixture is just blended (it should not be smooth), add pepper and salt to season. Set aside.

3. Meanwhile, fill the sous vide water oven and preheat to 144 degrees.

4. Rub oil on the shanks before seasoning with pepper and salt. Place the seasoned shanks inside a cooking pouch (large). Add 2 sprigs of thyme into each pouch

before vacuum sealing. Place in the preheated sous vide water oven and allow to cook for forty-eight hours. Once done, drain the pouch juices into a covered bowl and set aside in the refrigerator. Transfer the shanks onto a platter, separate the meat from the bones, cover, and set aside.

5. Pour the reserved pouch juices in a saucepan and heat on medium. Stir and cook until reduced and thickened, then pour into a sauce pot. Stir in the glace and simmer on low. Once the sauce is thick enough that it sticks to a spoon, add in the lamb meat. Stir to combine, making sure the meat is evenly coated with the sauce.

6. Divide the meat into four equal portions. Place each lamb meat portion on a sheet of cling film. Then roll to form a tight cylindrical shape. Place all rolled lamb meats in the refrigerator to chill overnight.

7. Take the chilled lamb cylinders out of their wraps and set on a plate. Meanwhile, fill 3 separate bowls with panko crumbs, egg wash, and flour. Coat the lamb cylinders with the flour before dipping into egg wash.

Transfer into the bowl containing the panko crumbs and dredge, then place on a large plate.

8. Heat a deep fryer on high before adding the oil. Once the oil reaches 165 degrees, add the breaded lamb cylinders and cook until golden brown. Place on layers of paper towels to drain.

9. Serve lamb croquettes with the prepared salsa verde.

10. Enjoy.

Lamb with Cabbage and Potato Fondants

Ingredients:

Lamb:

- Salt, kosher (1/4 teaspoon)

- Pepper, freshly cracked (1/4 teaspoon)

- Lamb rump steaks, 8-oz. (4 pieces)

- Red currant jelly (2 tablespoons)

Cabbage:

- Leeks (2 pieces)

- Olive oil, extra virgin (3 tablespoons)

- Double cream (10 ounces)

- Mustard, whole grain (1 teaspoon)

- Cabbage head, Savoy (1 piece)

- Pancetta, smoked (7 ounces)

- Chicken stock, reduced sodium (8 ounces)

- Butter (2 tablespoons)

Potato fondants:

- Butter (10 tablespoons)

- Garlic cloves, peeled (3 pieces)

- Potatoes, Maris Piper (8 pieces)

- Chicken stock (14 ounces)

- Thyme sprig, fresh (1 piece)

Directions:

1. Fill the sous vide water oven before preheating to 135 degrees. Set the conventional oven to 395 degrees to preheat as well.

2. Peel the potatoes before slicing into equal-sized barrel/ cylindrical shapes. Place in a medium bowl.

3. Meanwhile, heat a roasting tray on high. Add the butter and allow to melt and foam before adding the potatoes. Cook for two to three minutes or until all sides are cooked through and golden brown.

4. Stir in the garlic as well as thyme. Pour in the chicken stock and mix well before transferring the roasting tray into the preheated conventional oven. Cook for about forty-five minutes or until the potatoes are tender, moist, and cooked through.

5. Sprinkle pepper and steaks on the rump steaks before placing inside cooking pouches. Vacuum seal and place in the preheated sous vide water oven and allow to cook for forty-five minutes to one hour.

6. Discard the cabbage's outer leaves and hard stalk before slicing into fine shreds. Set aside in a small bowl.

7. Meanwhile, heat a frying pan on medium. Add oil and allow to get extremely hot before adding the pancetta. Cook until nicely crisp and golden. Stir in the butter; once foaming, stir in the cabbage and leeks as well. Sprinkle pepper and salt and fry for about three to four more minutes or until the cabbage and leeks are softened and a bit golden.

8. Pour in the stock. Allow the mixture to cook for an additional five minutes or until the leeks and cabbage and cooked through and tender. Add the mustard and double cream, then cook for another five minutes or until the mixture is reduced to ¾ its original volume. Cover to keep warm.

9. Once the rump steaks are done, remove from the sous vide water oven and transfer onto a plate. Pat dry with paper towels and set aside.

10. In the meantime, heat a pan on high. Once extremely hot, add the rump steaks and cook until both sides are browned. Place on a platter and set aside.

11. Turn the heat of the same pan down to low before adding in the currant jelly. Allow to melt and then

brush on the rump steaks, making sure all sides are evenly coated. Cut the glazed rump steaks to form 8 slices.

12. Divide the cabbage among 4 plates. Top each with 2 rump steak slices and serve alongside the potato fondants.

13. Enjoy.

9 - Delicious Sous Vide Duck for Dinner Recipes

Duck Breast with Farro and Blackberry Jam

Ingredients:

Duck breast:

- Thyme leaves, fresh, picked (1/2 tablespoon)

- Black pepper, freshly ground (1/4 teaspoon)

- Red onions, julienned (1 cup)

- Salt, kosher (1/4 teaspoon)

- Garlic clove, peeled, smashed (1 piece)

- Parsley, chopped (1 tablespoon)

- Duck breasts, 8-oz. (2 pieces)

- Thyme sprigs, fresh, divided (4 pieces)

- Olive oil, extra virgin (1 tablespoon)

- Brown sugar (1 tablespoon)

- Baby escarole heads, cut, washed (3 pieces)

- Shallots, minced (1 teaspoon)

- Farro, cooked (1 cup) – see below

Farro:

- Olive oil, extra virgin (1 tablespoon)

- Stock, chicken/ duck (2 cups)

- Carrot, peeled, diced finely (1/2 piece)

- Salt, kosher (1 teaspoon)

- Farro (3/4 cup)

- Celery stalk, trimmed, diced finely (1/2 piece)

- Turnip, peeled, diced finely (1/4 piece)

Blackberry jam:

- Sugar, granulated (3/4 cup)

- Blackberries, fresh (1 ¼ pounds)

- Lemon juice, freshly squeezed (1/2 tablespoon)

Directions:

1. Place the berries in a colander and rinse under cool water. Transfer into a large bowl and toss gently with sugar. Over the bowl and place in the refrigerator; allow the berries to marinate overnight. Heat a large saucepan over medium. Then add the marinated berries to warm and soften. Remove the seeds with a food mill/ fine-mesh sieve before returning to the pan. Heat on medium, cook until thickened and keep warm.

2. Heat a saucepan on medium-high. Add the farro and cook until lightly toasted. Stir in the oil, carrot, celery, and turnip; cook for two minutes or until a bit tender. Pour in the water and add in salt. Stir to combine and allow the mixture to boil before reducing heat to medium-low. Cover and simmer for half an hour or until a small amount of liquid remains. Once done, fluff the farro with a fork and set aside.

3. Heat a saucepan on medium-high before adding the oil (1 tablespoon). Once heated through, stir in the onions. Arrange the onions into an even layer before

sprinkling the brown sugar on top. Stir and cook until the onions are tender and browned, then place in a covered bowl and refrigerate.

4. Fill the sous vide water oven and preheat to 132 degrees.

5. Sprinkle black pepper on the duck breasts before placing inside a cooking pouch. Add a thyme sprig on top of each duck breast. Vacuum seal the cooking pouch before submerging in the sous vide water oven. Allow the duck breasts to cook for thirty minutes to two hours. Once done, remove from the cooking pouch and transfer onto a plate; pat dry with paper towels, season with salt, and set aside. Meanwhile, pour the pouch juices into a small bowl and reserve.

6. Heat a large sauté pan on medium before adding the olive oil. Once heated through, stir in the garlic clove as well as the rest of the thyme sprigs. Once the oil starts smoking, turn heat down to low and add the duck breasts. Cook with their skin sides down for seven minutes. Once the fat is rendered, pour it off the pan. Flip the duck breasts on the other side to

cook for an additional minute. Once done, place on a platter, cover, and let sit.

7. Discard the fat from the pan and return to the stove. Heat on medium-high before adding the escarole. Cook until caramelized and a bit wilted. Then pour in the reserved pouch juices. Add the farro and caramelized onions as well as the shallots and garlic; stir and cook until the entire mixture is warmed through. Stir in thyme and parsley before covering to keep warm.

8. Drizzle the prepared blackberry sauce on the plate to form streaks. Place a small mound of farro and escarole mixture on one side, and top with the sliced duck breast. Add fresh thyme leaves and serve immediately.

Peking Style Duck Legs and Eggs

Ingredients:

Duck legs:

- Duck fat (8 tablespoons)

- Duck legs (8 pieces)

- Oil, high smoke point – for deep frying

Duck eggs:

- Duck eggs (6 pieces)

Cucumber spaghetti:

- Soya sauce, dark (2 teaspoons)

- Ginger, fresh, grated finely (1 teaspoon)

- Sesame oil (1 tablespoon)

- Cucumber (1 piece)

- Balsamic vinegar (2 teaspoons)

- Garlic clove, peeled, grated finely (1 piece)

Spring onion puree:

- Onions, Spanish, peeled, sliced finely (3 pieces)

- Spring onions, green, washed, sliced thinly (6
  bunches)

- Pomace oil (2 tablespoons)

- Double cream (10 ounces)

- Salt, kosher (1/4 teaspoon)

Dressing:

- Honey (1/4 cup)

- Soya sauce, dark (1/4 cup)

- Sesame oil (1 tablespoon)

- Ketchup (8 ounces)

- Orange juice, freshly squeezed (1/4 cup)

- Oyster sauce (1/4 cup)

Pancake crumb:

- Salt, kosher (1/4 teaspoon)

- Pastry sheets, feuille de brick, torn into bits (3 pieces)

Directions:

1. Fill the sous vide water oven before preheating to 180 degrees.

2. Fill 2 cooking pouches (large) with the duck legs (4 legs into 1 pouch). Pour in the duck fat before vacuum sealing the pouches, then place in the sous vide water oven. Allow the duck legs to cook for twelve hours.

3. Once the dusk legs are done, remove from the pouches and place on top of paper towels to drain off excess fat. Separate the meat (while still warm) from the bone and shred into thin strips before placing in a covered bowl. Set aside.

4. Turn the sous vide water oven temperature down to 147 degrees. Gently submerge the duck eggs to cook for one hour and ten minutes.

5. Meanwhile, heat a saucepan on medium before adding pomace oil; spread to form a thin film on the pan surface. Stir in the Spanish onions as well as salt (a pinch). Allow the onions to sweat for about four to five minutes or until translucent and softened.

6. Stir in the cream before turning the heat up to medium-high and allowing the mixture to boil. Stir in the spring onions; cook for about two to three minutes or until tender. Pour the mixture into the

blender and process until well-combined and smooth. Transfer the puree to a large bowl and place in the refrigerator.

7. After peeling and deseeding the cucumber, cut into long, extremely thin strands. Place in a large bowl and set aside.

8. Place all the ingredients for the cucumber strands in a small bowl. Stir to combine and set aside (toss with the cucumber later). Do the same with the ingredients for preparing the duck dressing.

9. Heat a deep fryer before adding the oil. Once the oil is heated to 356 degrees, add the shredded duck leg and cook until crispy. Once done, transfer onto a plate lined with paper towels and set aside.

10. Add pastry pieces to the same heated oil. Cook for half a minute, drain, and season with a bit of salt. Set aside.

11. Heat the pureed spring onion until warmed through, then divide among 4 plates. Gently toss the crispy duck meat with ½ of the dressing; divide among 4

portions and place each onto one plate (on top of the pureed spring onion).

12. Finish each plate by adding one duck egg, ¼ of the dressed cucumber strands, ¼ of the pancake crumbs, and ¼ of the remaining duck dressing.

13. Serve and enjoy.

Juniper Berry Duck

Ingredients:

- Thyme sprigs, fresh (3 pieces)

- Juniper berries, fresh-dried, red raisin (1/2 cup)

- Duck leg, quarter (1 piece)

- Salt, kosher (1/4 teaspoon)

- Spinach, fresh (1 cup)

- Orange zest, freshly grated (1 tablespoon)

- Orange fruit (1 piece)

Directions:

1. Fill the sous vide water oven before preheating to 165 degrees.

2. Place the duck leg in a large bowl. Rub salt all over its sides before setting aside.

3. Use a vegetable peeler to strip off the zest from the orange. Section the fruit and place in a small bowl.

4. Place the juniper berries on a sheet of cling film. Top with the orange zest as well as thyme sprigs before loosely rolling. Place inside a small cooking pouch (quart size) and then top with a layer of orange sections. Add the salted duck leg in the middle before vacuum sealing the pouch.

5. Squeeze the orange pieces through the pouch before dropping the pouch into the sous vide water oven. Cook the duck leg for five to eight hours.

6. Once the duck leg is done, remove from the sous vide water oven. Drain the pouch juices into a skillet; set aside.

7. Meanwhile, set the broiler on high to preheat.

8. Unroll the juniper berry wrap and transfer the contents into the skillet containing the pouch juices. Heat on medium and cook the mixture until reduced. Season with pepper and salt, remove from heat and set aside.

9. Place the cooked duck leg below the preheated broiler to sear. Once done, transfer onto a platter.

10. Serve the broiled duck leg alongside a mound of fresh spinach. Smother with orange sauce and enjoy.

Easy Seared Duck

Ingredients:

- Shallots, chopped (2 tablespoons)

- Broccoli stalks, Chinese (2 pieces)

- Duck breasts, 8-oz. (4 pieces)

- Red wine (2 tablespoons)

Marinade:

- Cinnamon sticks (2 pieces)

- Tong kwai herb (4 pieces)

- Sugar (1 teaspoon)

- Spring onions, green (2 pieces)

- Star anise pods (2 pieces)

- Ginger, fresh, minced (2 coins)

- Garlic cloves, peeled, mashed (4 pieces)

- Salt, kosher (1 teaspoon)

Ginger water:

- Water, filtered (3 ¼ ounces)

- Sugar (1/2 teaspoon)

- Ginger, sliced (3 ¼ ounces)

- Rice wine, Chinese (3 ¼ ounces)

- Salt, kosher (1/2 teaspoon)

Reduction base:

- Chicken, roasted (1/2 piece)

- Oyster sauce (2 teaspoons)

- Onion, large, peeled, sliced, sautéed (1/4 piece)

- Soy sauce, light (5 ounces)

- Chicken stock, reduced sodium (5 ounces)

- Apple, large, peeled, sliced, sautéed (1/4 piece)

Directions:

1. Place the duck breast inside a cooking pouch. Add the ingredients for the marinade before vacuum sealing and placing in the refrigerator to marinate overnight.

2. Fill the sous vide water oven and preheat to 133 degrees.

3. Add the duck breast pouch into the sous vide water oven and cook for fifty minutes.

4. Pour water into the blender. Add the ginger and process until well-combined into a paste. Pass the ginger paste through a sieve and set aside the liquid in a small bowl.

5. Fill a saucepan with the Chinese wine. Add the re-

served ginger liquid and stir to combine. Stir in the salt and sugar before heating the saucepan on medium-high. Allow the mixture to boil and then set aside.

6. Pour the ingredients for the reduction base into a pot. Stir to combine, heat on medium-high, and allow the mixture to simmer for an hour or until reduced to 2/3 its original volume. Pour into a sieve set atop a medium bowl; set aside.

7. Fill a pot with water and heat on medium-high. Once boiling, add the gai lan yo blanch for one minute. Remove and set aside in a small bowl.

8. Heat a skillet on medium-high before adding the shallots. Once fragrant, pour in the red wine as well as reduction base (100 milliliters). Stir and cook until the mixture is reduced to 2/3 its original amount. Remove from heat and set aside.

9. Meanwhile, heat a skillet on medium. Add the duck breast and cook until seared and browned on both sides. Once done, transfer to a plate.

10. Serve the duck leg alongside the blanched gai lan and topped with the reduction sauce.

Ginger Garlic Duck Breasts

Ingredients:

- Ginger garlic paste (4 teaspoons)

- Shallots, peeled (6 ounces)

- Coriander powder, ground (2 teaspoons)

- Coconut milk (3 ½ ounces)

- Salt, kosher (1/4 teaspoon)

- Coconut oil (1 teaspoon)

- Raisins (12 pieces)

- Tomato sauce (14 ½ ounces)

- Duck breasts (2 pieces)

- Turmeric (1 teaspoon)

- Curry leaves (2 stems)

- Cashew nuts, halved (2 pieces)

- Chili powder, Kashmiri (2 teaspoons)

- Garam masala (1/2 teaspoon)

- Onions, caramelized (1/2 cup)

Directions:

1. Trim the fat layers off the duck breasts before scoring the meats. Place in a large bowl and set aside.

2. Place ginger garlic paste (1 teaspoon) in a medium bowl. Add turmeric powder and salt, then stir well to combine. Pour the mixture onto the duck breasts, turning the latter to coat evenly on all sides. Cover and place in the refrigerator to marinate for thirty minutes.

3. Fill the sous vide water oven before preheating to 140 degrees.

4. Remove the marinated duck breasts from the refrigerator and transfer into a large cooking pouch. Vacuum seal before submerging in the preheated sous vide water oven. Allow the duck breasts to cook for

two hours and thirty minutes.

5. Meanwhile, heat a pan (heavy bottomed) on medium before adding the coconut oil. Once the oil is heated through, add the sliced shallots as well as curry leaves; sauté until golden brown.

6. Stir in the raisins, cashew nut, and the rest of the ground spices and ginger garlic paste. Cook for an additional minute before adding in the duck breast. Cook until the surfaces are nicely seared.

7. Pour in the tomato sauce as well as a small amount of water. Stir and allow the mixture to simmer until thickened, before stirring in the salt and coconut milk.

8. Serve the duck meat over a pool of ginger garlic sauce. Top with caramelized onions and enjoy.

10 - Conclusion

Now you know everything there is to know about cooking your food the sous vide way, so any misgivings you may have about giving it a go should be tossed out the kitchen window.

Not sure about the safety of cooking bags or pouches used to hold your ingredients? Rest assured that sous vide plastic containers are made of inert polyethylene material, which means that it does not contain harmful substances like phthalate or BPA that can leach into your "sous videlicious" fares.

You do have to be extra careful with refrigerating your sous vide cooked food. Once you open the pouch, make sure to consume the contents right away or within three days. Sticking your sous vide cooked food in the refrigerator for more than that time frame only gives bacteria the opportunity to flourish and cause you potential harm.

Don't get yourself tied up in choosing the most digitally enhanced sous vide immersion circulator or water oven. The point of cooking with the sous vide method is to be able to cook your food perfectly each and every time after setting your cooking device to your target time and temperature.

Your immersion circulator or water oven can be left alone to work on your food and give you the exact results you want, even if you don't adjust the controls.

Lastly, give yourself a chance to breathe and relax in the knowledge that it is perfectly fine if it takes you several tries before achieving perfection. Once you master the sous vide method of cooking your favorite dishes, eating gourmet quality food at home every day and night of your life is possible.

Book 4 - Sous Vide

Ultimate Low-Temperature Immersion Circulator Guide
(Modern Technique, Step-by-Step Instructions, Cooking
Through Science)

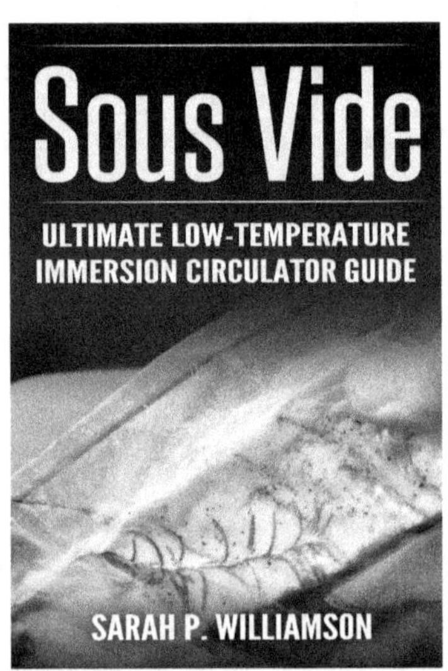

1 - Introduction

Deceptively Easy

On the outside, it looks intimidating, but the truth is that sous vide cooking is downright simple and achievable. The term "sous vide" is French for "under vacuum" and is used in modern cooking to mean vacuum-sealing your food and then bathing them in warm water for a specific period of time.

This cooking method gives you flavorful food without being overcooked. The food also brims with aromas and juices that make it seem like you are serving up restaurant-quality dishes in the comfort of your home.

Long History

Cooking the sous vide way has a long history of being part of modernist cuisine.

- 1960s: American and French engineers discovered that placing meat inside vacuum bags before cooking them at low temperatures give a more wonderfully textured meat as opposed to cooking it through traditional means.

- 1970s: Top restaurants all over the world started using the sous vide method of cooking to turn out superior quality dishes.

- 1990s: Food scientists performed extensive studies on the sous vide way of cooking food.

- The late 2000s: Sous vide cooking found its way into home kitchens.

- 2008: Thomas Keller, a renowned chef, introduced a guide to the sous vide cooking technique and paved the way for sous vide to be widely used in many U.S. restaurants.

- Present: Both high-end food establishments and home kitchens are serving up meals that are cooked the sous vide way.

Within Reach

The sous vide cooking technique is now more accessible than ever, thanks to immersion circulators that are commercially available in varying sizes, ease of use, and costs. Much of the equipment is handy enough to store inside your kitchen drawer, with some of them being practically a no-brainer with the app-controlled interfaces they come with.

But having a high-tech and ultra-streamlined immersion circulator at your disposal does not mean you have no need of other sous vide equipment. You still need a container to hold your water bath in, a requirement that a twelve-quart cooking pot might easily fill.

But you can choose from plenty of plastic food storage containers that allow you to easily monitor your food as it cooks in the water bath; plus, these commercial food containers possess superior heat retention capabilities.

You also need a vacuum sealer to secure your food in their bags – you can use Ziploc bags if you prefer to cut down on cost, although making use of specially designed plastic bags and securing them with a vacuum sealer allows you to reduce your risk of error and increase your chances of cooking perfect meals.

2 - Sous Videlicious Benefits

The fact that sous vide cooking allows you to accurately control cooking temperatures means that you also get to enjoy these benefits:

You are assured that your food is cooked with consistent doneness from the edges to the center.

You have the opportunity to recreate your meals with near-perfection.

You have greater control on your food's level of doneness, something that is difficult to achieve when cooking through conventional methods.

You can pasteurize your food to make it safe for eating even when cooked at low temperatures (your sous vide steak is safe to eat even when not cooked well-done and your tougher meat cuts can turn out tender even when cooked medium-rare).

You will look forward to getting perfect results each and every time you cook. Cooking chicken breasts, steaks, and other fast-cooking food the sous vide way lets you enjoy the process of cooking itself because you are no longer preoccupied with the usual guesswork that comes with cooking food by traditional means.

When you cook your food using the sous vide technique, thermometer-poking, finger-jabbing, and cutting-and-peeking will now be things of the past.

You enjoy a more flexible schedule that lets you fit in other important tasks. As your immersion circulator quietly heats the bath in which your vacuum-sealed food is submerged in the kitchen, gradually softening your meat until medium-rare and perfectly succulent, you are able to work on your household chores, baby tasks, or exercise routines.

You have the option to pre-cook (long enough to ensure the food is pasteurized) your food (see to it that they are fresh and free from contamination), then chill in the ice bath (for forty-five minutes) before placing in the freezer. Later, you simply reheat, serve, and enjoy eating them.

Know that your sous vide cooked food will always turn out perfectly if you make sure to reheat them below their target cooking temperatures. The one thing you need to keep in mind is the possibility of food contamination, which is why following all the cooking procedures is crucial to guarantee food safety.

(In case there are steps you are not that confident with, it would be best to just eat the sous vide cooked food right away.)

3 - Sous Vide Elements

Sous vide cooking consists of these three elements:

Vacuum sealing

Vacuum sealing your food for sous vide cooking results in the efficient transfer of heat from water bath to your food. This helps in preventing any loss of aromas and juices through evaporation during cooking. Because your ingredients are enclosed in the vacuum-sealed bag along with their accompanying spices/herbs, the latter are able to deliver added flavor in a more intense manner.

Ensuring that your food are vacuum sealed for sous vide cooking also helps in avoiding any off-flavors that might result from the oxidation process (an example would be your meat's fat becoming rancid after long periods of exposure to air).

Moreover, vacuum sealing your sous vide ingredients helps in reducing the risk of re-contaminating them while they are in storage, especially if you are going to cook, store (refrigerate or freeze), and reheat.

Cooking at precise temperatures

Cooking at precise temperatures, an important feature of the sous vide cooking method, allows you to avoid cooking mishaps that can range from turning your should-have-been-perfectly-poached eggs into a single, runny mess, to turning your would-have-been-tender-and-flavorful chicken breast or fish fillet into an ugly, mushy mass.

Cooking at exact times and temperatures also ensures that your food is safe for consumption and helps you figure out its expected shelf life. Because the sous vide cooking method was created with the help of science, you are assured that you will be able to cook your food with perfect timing and with the exact temperature each and every time.

Cooking at low temperatures

At the heart of sous vide cooking is the idea that heat is transferred more effectively through water than through air. This is why you are better off cooking your steak at 135 degrees Fahrenheit in the water bath instead of cooking it at 350 degrees Fahrenheit in a conventional oven.

Besides, cooking at low temperatures lets you turn out more

succulent results. This is because low cooking temperatures do not cause the cell walls in your meat to burst; instead, their connective tissues' tough collagen parts get hydrolyzed into a gelatinous mass.

(In traditional cooking with high temperatures, the same collagen would have been overheated to the point that they are too denatured, resulting in your meat becoming tougher and depleted of moisture, which equals zero flavor.) You can also rest assured that cooking your vegetables at sous vide low temperatures lets you cook them thoroughly and still get that crisp and firm texture you desire.

4 - Sous Vide Prepping Pointers

Preparing your food for cooking the sous vide way is as easy as 1, 2, 3, 4!

Portioning the food

It is best to cut your food into small portions first before cooking with the sous vide method. Doing so ensures that the food reaches the target temperature more quickly and will be cooked through the center.

It is important to see to it that your food gets cooked as quickly as possible, especially when it comes to fish and other extremely tender food – they tend to get mushy when submerged too long in a warm bath.

Another advantage to cutting your food into small portions before sous vide cooking is that you prevent any large areas from being in the dangerous temperature range (40 degrees to 140 degrees Fahrenheit) for long periods, in which microbial spoilage can occur.

Seasoning the food

Generously season your food with pepper and salt as well as your preferred spices and herbs.

Bagging and vacuum sealing the food

When cooking large batches of food, or when finding it difficult to place awkwardly-shaped ingredients inside the usual zip-top plastic bags, you can use special vacuum bags that are ideal for sous vide cooking. You can rely on these bags to stand up to tears, leaks, high cooking temperatures, and freezing.

Cooking the food

When cooking your food the sous vide way, you are basically submerging it in the water bath that is preheated to your target temperature. Water is known to be a better conductor of heat than air. Add in the immersion circulator and you are assured that all areas of your water bath is evenly heated.

Cooking your food with the sous vide technique allows you to serve up foods that are evenly cooked through, thanks to the fact that the temperature outside is equal to your target cooking temperature. Another great thing about sous vide cooking is that even if you let your food remain in the bath beyond its targeted time, it will not get overcooked as the temperature will remain constant.

Finishing the food

Once your food is done being sous vide cooked, you can serve it immediately – simply open the vacuum sealed bag, remove the food, and transfer it onto a serving plate. Sous vide cooked foods appear poached when served, which means you can usually serve eggs, skinless poultry meats, fish, and shellfish as is.

As for other meats like steak, lamb, and pork, these are not usually served poached, so you can make them look even more palatable by searing after cooking.

A great steak is usually characterized by a wonderfully browned and seared surface. Most of the steak's flavor comes from this tasty, crispy skin, something that you can get only if you subject it to high temperatures. Now, sous vide cooking is all about cooking your food at low temperature, so it is important to sear the food afterwards to make sure it develops that much desired browned taste.

You may use a blowtorch to sear smaller cuts of meat. A blowtorch's high heat effectively sears food surfaces while leaving the interior of the sliced parts alone. To prevent any unpleasant aromas that might result from searing your food with a blowtorch, make sure to use the recommended MAPP (methylacetylene propadiene propene) gas.

If searing flat sous vide cooked foods, there is always the pan or griddle to help you. You can sear chicken, pork, or beef in a pan made of cast iron, and fish, scallops, and other more delicate foods in a pan made of stainless steel.

To get the temperature transfer going at a faster rate, you can grease the pan first with a high smoke point oil like sunflower oil or canola oil. Heat the pan before adding about a tablespoon of oil (just enough to coat the entire pan's bottom). Once the oil is hot, smoking, and starting to brown, add the sous vide cooked meat (pat-dried with paper towels).

You may also use an extremely hot grill to give your sous vide cooked foods those desired grill marks.

If you wish to deep fry your sous vide cooked foods for a deeply browned and crispier exterior, try dipping them first in liquid nitrogen; this will help keep the foods from being overcooked as they are deep-fried.

5 - Quick Guide to Sous Vide Tools

Things to Consider

Temperature stability

Any change in temperature by as much as one degree makes a huge difference to how your sous vide cooked food turns out. Make sure to use are using a sous vide tool that possesses a ± 32 degrees Fahrenheit temperature stability. Due to its water pumps and other electronics, using an immersion circulator will ensure that the water in your bath is circulated properly.

Water bath container

Choose a water bath container that is specially manufactured for use in sous vide cooking. This will assure you of excellent insulation for less energy consumption as well as reduced water evaporation, which are crucial when cooking your food for more than eighteen hours.

Water bath capacity

You can choose water bath containers with capacities that range from 5 liters to 120 liters. The important thing to remember is that you have to have adequate free space between all food bags you place inside the water bath – this is to ensure that the water can circulate well. Make sure not to fill more than ½ of the water bath container with food bags.

Heating power

The heating power of your immersion circulator determines the time it takes to heat up your water bath to reach the target temperature before cooking the food.

Size of equipment

Immersion circulators are handy and take up only a small space in your kitchen. You can even store them standing up on the counter, which is great for keeping your kitchen clutter-free and organized-looking.

Maintenance and cleaning

Make sure to choose sous vide tools that are easy to clean, easy to maintain, have no exposed parts to cause you harm, and if possible, coated with nonstick surfaces.

Safety

One concern with sous vide cooking is the fact that you are dealing with evaporating water. This is the reason you need to make sure that your sous vide cooking bags are properly and constantly submerged in the heated water bath. Look for a device that has a lid to ensure decreased water evaporation.

You might also try a device that comes with an alarm that gets triggered whenever the water level measuring part of the device detects an extremely low water level. It would also be best to make sure that your immersion circulator comes with a protective shield for helping keep the sous vide bags away from the pump and heating coil.

6 - Essentials to Have

Aside from sous vide cooking bags to place your food in, you need the following:

Immersion circulator

An immersion circulator comes with motors that heat the water in your bath, and then circulate it inside the container. This is what keeps the temperature of the water constant and evenly distributed, both of which are important in sous vide cooking.

What is great about using an immersion circulator is that you can use it with different sizes of cooking pots. This device is also small enough to be easily stored, always a plus when choosing any kitchen device.

Vacuum sealer (chamber vacuum packer)

A chamber vacuum packer or sealer lets you seal your sous vide food bags with ease and peace of mind. Simply position the whole cooking bag inside the inner chamber of the machine. Close the lid and allow the packer to extract the air inside the chamber, which forces out the air from inside the bag.

Thermometer

A thermometer of good quality, when used with a special foam tape, is useful in monitoring your food's temperature once it is placed in the sous vide bag. This is important because it gives you an idea of when your food will reach its target temperature for cooking perfectly.

7 - Tips on Sous Vide Target Times and Temperatures

Steak: T-Bone/Porterhouse, Ribeye, Butcher's Cuts, and Strip

The following timings are provided for steaks cut that are about 1½-inches to 2-inches thick. If cooking steaks with a thickness of 1-inch or less, you can shorten the initial cooking time to forty minutes. For steaks that are sous vide cooked at less than 130 degrees Fahrenheit, make sure to cook them for no more than 2½ hours to keep them safe for consumption.

Very rare/Rare doneness

- Temperature range – 120 degrees Fahrenheit to 128 degrees Fahrenheit

- Timing range – 1 hour to 2 hours

Medium to rare doneness

- Temperature range – 129 degrees Fahrenheit to 134 degrees Fahrenheit

- Timing range – 1 hour to 4 hours (if under 130 degrees Fahrenheit, it should be 2 ½ hours maximum)

Medium doneness

- Temperature range – 135 degrees Fahrenheit to 144 degrees Fahrenheit

- Timing range – 1 hour to 4 hours

Medium to well-done

- Temperature range – 145 degrees Fahrenheit to 155 degrees Fahrenheit

- Timing range – 1 hour to 3 ½ hours

Well-done

- Temperature range – 156 degrees Fahrenheit and up

- Timing range – 1 hour to 3 hours

Steak: Tenderloin

It is easy to overcook lean tenderloin and have it end up dry because of the absence of intramuscular fat in this cut of meat. To avoid this dilemma, consider cooking your tenderloin at a temperature that is several Fahrenheit degrees lower than ribeye, strip, and other fattier meat cuts.

You might also try sous vide cooking your tenderloin between very rare and rare (within 120 degrees Fahrenheit and 128 degrees Fahrenheit) to ensure that it is tenderly cooked and retains its juiciness.

The following timings are for steaks that are about 1 ½ to 2 inches in thickness. If cooking steaks with 1 inch or less thickness, simply decrease the initial cooking time to thirty minutes. If cooking steaks below 130 degrees Fahrenheit, see to it that you cook it for more than 2 ½ hours to ensure food safety.

Very rare/Rare doneness

- Temperature range – 120 degrees Fahrenheit to 128 degrees Fahrenheit

- Timing range – 45 minutes to 2 ½ hours

Medium to rare doneness

- Temperature range – 129 degrees Fahrenheit to 134 degrees Fahrenheit

- Timing range – 45 minutes to 4 hours (if under 130

degrees Fahrenheit, it should be 2 ½ hours maximum)

Medium doneness

- Temperature range – 135 degrees Fahrenheit to 144
degrees Fahrenheit

- Timing range – 45 minutes to 4 hours

Medium to well-done

- Temperature range – 145 degrees Fahrenheit to 155
degrees Fahrenheit

- Timing range – 45 minutes to 3 ½ hours

Well-done

- Temperature range – 156 degrees Fahrenheit and up

- Timing range – 1 hour to 3 hours

Chicken Breast

Tender and juicy – great for using in cold chicken salads

- Temperature range – 150 degrees Fahrenheit

- Timing range – 1 hour to 4 hours

Juicy and very soft – best served hot

- Temperature range – 140 degrees Fahrenheit

- Timing range – 1 ½ hours to 4 hours

Slightly stringy, tender, and juicy – best served hot

- Temperature range – 150 degrees Fahrenheit

- Timing range – 1 hour to 4 hours

Slightly stringy, traditional, firm, and juicy – best served hot

- Temperature range – 160 degrees Fahrenheit

- Timing range – 1 hour to 4 hours

Shrimp

Translucent, semi-raw, and with buttery, soft texture

- Temperature range – 125 degrees Fahrenheit

- Timing range – 15 minutes

Nearly opaque, slightly firm, very tender

- Temperature range – 130 degrees Fahrenheit

- Timing range – 15 minutes

Barely opaque, juicy, tender, and moist

- Temperature range – 135 degrees Fahrenheit

- Timing range – 15 minutes

Poached texture, traditional, juicy, with good bounce, and with snappy bite

- Temperature range – 140 degrees Fahrenheit

- Timing range – 15 minutes

Lobster

Translucent and soft

- Temperature range – 120 degrees Fahrenheit

- Timing range – 20 minutes

Succulent and tender

- Temperature range – 130 degrees Fahrenheit

- Timing range – 30 minutes to 45 minutes

Traditional, with steamed lobster texture

- Temperature range – 140 degrees Fahrenheit

- Timing range – 1 hour

Halibut

Tender, just about to flake, and with near-raw layers

- Temperature range – 125 degrees Fahrenheit

- Timing range – 45 minutes for 1-inch thick fillets; 45 minutes to 1 hour for up to 2-inches thick fillets

Tender, flaky, and extremely moist

- Temperature range – 130 degrees Fahrenheit

- Timing range – 45 minutes for 1-inch thick fillets; 45 minutes to 1 hour for up to 2-inches thick fillets

Firm, flaky, moist, and about to develop a tough texture

- Temperature range – 140 degrees Fahrenheit

- Timing range – 45 minutes for 1-inch thick fillets; 45 minutes to 1 hour for up to 2-inches thick fillets

Tuna

Rare/nearly raw, slightly firm, to be served chilled

- Temperature range – 105 degrees Fahrenheit

- Timing range – 45 minutes for 1-inch thick fillets; 45 minutes to 1 hour for up to 2-inches thick fillets

Just firmed and extremely moist

- Temperature range – 110 degrees Fahrenheit

- Timing range – 45 minutes for 1-inch thick fillets; 45 minutes to 1 hour for up to 2-inches thick fillets

Moist and meaty

- Temperature range – 115 degrees Fahrenheit

- Timing range – 45 minutes for 1-inch thick fillets; 45 minutes to 1 hour for up to 2-inches thick fillets

Dry, firm, and with well-done steak texture

- Temperature range – 120 degrees Fahrenheit

- Timing range – 45 minutes for 1-inch thick fillets; 45 minutes to 1 hour for up to 2-inches thick fillets

Firm, crumbly, dry, and to be used in recipes calling for canned tuna

- Temperature range – 130 degrees Fahrenheit

- Timing range – 45 minutes for 1-inch thick fillets; 45 minutes to 1 hour for up to 2-inches thick fillets

Lamb

Very rare/rare doneness

- Temperature range – 115 degrees Fahrenheit to 124 degrees Fahrenheit

- Timing range – 1 hour to 4 hours (if cooking under 130 degrees Fahrenheit, it should be 2 ½ hours maximum)

Medium to rare doneness

- Temperature range – 125 degrees Fahrenheit to 134

degrees Fahrenheit

- Timing range – 45 minutes to 4 hours (if cooking under 130 degrees Fahrenheit, it should be 2 ½ hours maximum)

Medium doneness

- Temperature range – 135 degrees Fahrenheit to 144 degrees Fahrenheit

- Timing range – 1 hour to 4 hours

Medium to well-done

- Temperature range – 145 degrees Fahrenheit to 154 degrees Fahrenheit

- Timing range – 1 hour to 4 hours

Well-done

- Temperature range – 155 degrees Fahrenheit and up

- Timing range – 1 hour to 4 hours

Turkey

Very pink, extra moist, and soft

- Temperature range – 132 degrees Fahrenheit / 130 degrees Fahrenheit

- Timing range – 2 hours / 4 hours

Pale pink, moist, and soft

- Temperature range – 138 degrees Fahrenheit / 136 degrees Fahrenheit

- Timing range – 1 hour / 3 hours

White, moist, and tender

- Temperature range – 145 degrees Fahrenheit / 143 degrees Fahrenheit

- Timing range – 16 minutes / 2 ½ hours

White, with traditional roasted texture

- Temperature range – 152 degrees Fahrenheit / 150 degrees Fahrenheit

- Timing range – 4 minutes / 2 hours

8 - Guide to Sous Vide Cooking Steak

Step-by-Step Instructions for Sous Vide Cooking Steak:

1. Set the sous vide cooker to the target temperature to preheat. Add the steak only once the desired temperature is reached by the water bath.

2. Sprinkle the steak generously with pepper and salt, making sure the edges are seasoned as well, before placing in the cooking pouch or bag.

3. Add in any aromatics you want to use in your steak, such as sprigs of rosemary or thyme. See to it that they are evenly distributed on both surfaces of the seasoned steak.

4. Seal the cooking bag using a vacuum sealer or through the displacement method (if cooking your steak in a bag with a zipper-lock). If using the displacement method, gradually lower the cooking bag into a pot filled with water, then allow water pressure to press out the air inside the bag through its top. Securely seal the bag over the waterline as soon as most

of the air pockets are released.

5. Place the steak bag in the preheated water bath and allow it to sink. Follow the correct timing in cooking the steak.

6. Once the steak is done, remove the cooking bag out of the sous vide cooker. Take the steak out of the bag and transfer onto a plate lined with paper towels. To dry, carefully pat on both sides.

Step-by-Step Instructions for Finishing the Sous Vide Cooked Steak (Stovetop):

1. Heat a large cast iron skillet (heavy bottomed) over high heat. Add the vegetable oil (1 tablespoon), turning the skillet to spread the oil evenly.

2. Once the oil is heated through and is beginning to smoke, add the steak as well as butter (1 tablespoon), if preferred, to help the steak develop a dark crust and slightly charred taste.

3. Add whole sprigs of rosemary and thyme to the pan, as well as crushed garlic cloves and sliced shallots.

4. Allow the steak to cook for fifteen to thirty seconds on one side, then flip it every fifteen seconds thereafter in the next one minutes and thirty seconds or until nicely browned and seared. If you skipped the butter earlier, add it to the pan about half a minute before the steak is cooked.

5. Give your sous vide steak that steakhouse-quality char by flaming with a torch (high output). Avoid any off-aromas from the torched steak by making sure to simultaneously heat it in the skillet. Use slow and even strokes in torching on one side, making sure to apply the torch flame back and forth on the surface. Once the meat turns pale brown and shows several singed spots, flip to torch on the other side.

6. Use tongs to hold the steak by the edges. Rotate the meat on its edges as you cook it for an additional forty-five seconds or until all edges are browned.

7. Set a wire rack inside a baking sheet (rimmed). Once the steak is done, transfer to the rack and allow it to rest.

8. Serve the steak drenched in reheated pan juices and

fat.

Step-by-Step Instructions for Finishing the Sous Vide Cooked Steak (Grill):

1. Finishing your sous vide cooked steak on the grill will be a breeze if you do it outside. Place the cooked steak inside a cooler and bring outside.

2. Fill a chimney with lots of charcoal. Light the charcoal and allow it to burn until covered with ash. Discard the ash and set the coals to one corner of the grate. After setting the cooking grate into place, cover the grill and preheat for about five minutes.

3. Add the steak directly on top of the grill's hot side. Cook for about one minute and thirty seconds or until deeply crusted on the surface (make sure to turn the steak every fifteen to thirty seconds).

4. Once the steak is done, place on a platter. Serve and enjoy.

9 - Recipe Using Sous Vide Cooked Steak:

Salsa Verde Steak with Corn Salad

Ingredients:

Salsa verde:

- Cornichons, minced finely (8 pieces)

- Anchovy fillets, roughly minced (6 pieces)

- Olive oil, extra virgin (1/2 cup)

- Parsley leaves, fresh, minced (1 cup + 1 tablespoon)

- Dijon mustard (2 teaspoons)

- Sherry vinegar (2 tablespoons)

- Capers, drained, minced finely (2 tablespoons)

- Garlic cloves, medium, minced (2 pieces)

- Mint leaves, fresh, minced (1/2 cup + 1/2 tablespoon)

- Shallot, small, minced (2 tablespoons)

- Salt, kosher (1/2 teaspoon)

- Black pepper, freshly ground (1/2 teaspoon)

Salad:

- Steak, sous vide cooked, pan-seared, chilled, sliced thinly (3/4 pound)

- Corn ears, in husk (2 pieces)

- Red onion, sliced thinly (1 piece)

Directions:

1. Pour the sherry vinegar into a large mixing bowl. Add the anchovies, cornichons, parsley, shallot, capers, garlic, mint, and mustard. Whisk well to combine before drizzling in the olive oil. Season with pepper and salt; let sit.

2. Meanwhile, shuck the corn before grilling under the broiler or on top of a heated grill. Make sure to turn the corn frequently as it cooks for eight minutes or until tender and a bit charred. (You may also put the shucked corn on a plate (microwave safe) and microwave it for about seven minutes or until tender and steamed through.) Once the corn is done, let sit until slightly cooled and then cut off its kernels.

3. Discard the corn cobs, then place the corn kernels in a large mixing bowl. Add the red onion as well as steak and salsa verde (1/2 cup), then toss to combine. Season with pepper and salt before transferring the steak mixture onto a platter. Pour on some extra salsa verde and then top with mint and parsley leaves.

4. Serve right away.

5. Enjoy.

10 - Guide to Sous Vide Cooking Lamb

Step-by-Step Instructions for Sous Vide Cooking a Lamb Rack:

1. Set the sous vide cooker to your target temperature to preheat. (Once that temperature is reached, you can then add the lamb rack.)

2. Liberally season all sides of the lamb rack with pepper and salt.

3. Place the seasoned lamb rack inside the sous vide bag before vacuum sealing.

4. Submerge the lamb rack bag into the preheated water bath to cook.

5. Take the sous vide cooked lamb rack out of the bag and transfer onto a plate lined with paper towels. Carefully pat it dry on each side.

6. Heat a stainless steel/ cast iron skillet (heavy bottomed) on high, then add vegetable oil/ rice bran oil/ canola oil (1 tablespoon). Once the oil is smoking, add the lamb rack with the bones facing up and making

sure that the skillet is not crowded. To avoid this, consider cooking in batches.

7. Heat a cast iron skillet on medium-high. Add butter (1 tablespoon); once melted, add garlic cloves and shallot (roughly chopped) or whole sprigs of rosemary or thyme. Add the lamb and toss in the skillet so that all sides are evenly seared. Spoon the butter onto the lamb to baste it as it cooks for one minute. Turn the lamb to its other side and cook for an additional minute, making sure to baste it with butter as well.

8. Once the lamb is done, transfer to a cutting board. Use a sharp knife to slice down the ribs.

9. Serve smothered with the juices and fat left in the skillet.

Recipe Using Sous Vide Cooked Lamb:

Black Mustard and Mint Leg of Lamb

Ingredients:

- Black mustard seeds, whole (1 tablespoon)

- Mint leaves, fresh, chopped finely (1 ounce)

- Chili, red jalapeno/ Fresno, minced finely (1 piece)

- Salt, kosher (1/4 teaspoon)

- Black pepper, freshly ground (1/4 teaspoon)

- Shallot, small, minced (1 piece)

- Olive oil, extra virgin (3 tablespoons)

- Vegetable oil, divided (3 tablespoons)

- Cumin seeds, whole (2 teaspoons)

- Leg of lamb, boneless, butterflied, 5-pounds (1/2 piece)

- Cilantro leaves, fresh, w/ intact tender steams, chopped finely (1 ounce)

- Garlic clove, medium, minced finely (1 piece)

- Red wine vinegar (1 tablespoon)

Directions:

1. Heat a small skillet on medium-high, then add in the vegetable oil (2 tablespoons). Allow the oil to heat

through and shimmer before stirring in the cumin as well as the mustard. Cook for about half a minute or until fragrant; once done, pour right away into a large bowl (heat-proof), sprinkle with pepper and salt, and set aside to cool.

2. Take ½ portion of the cooled spice mixture and rub on the lamb leg's interior side. Roll back up and secure with a kitchen twine, making sure to tie from each end of the leg and working your way toward the middle at one-inch intervals. Season with additional pepper and salt before setting aside on a tray.

3. Meanwhile, set the water bath to the target temperature to preheat. Place the rolled lamb leg inside a sous vide bag, vacuum seal, and submerge in the water bath to cook until tenderly done.

4. Place the mustard-cumin mixture in a large bowl. Add the red wine vinegar as well as olive oil, garlic, cilantro, chili, mint, and shallot. Stir well to combine before adding in pepper and salt; let the chimichurri sit.

5. Once the lamb is done, remove from the sous vide

bag and transfer onto a large plate lined with paper towels. Pat dry carefully and set aside.

6. Heat a large skillet (cast iron) on medium before adding in vegetable oil (1 tablespoon). Once the oil is lightly smoking, add the sous vide cooked lamb and cook for about four minutes or until all of its sides are nicely browned.

7. Untie the twine off the lamb. Slice, serve and enjoy the prepared chimichurri.

11 - Guide to Sous Vide Cooking Chicken Breast

Step-by-Step Instructions for Sous Vide Cooking a Chicken Breast:

1. Set the sous vide cooker to your target temperature.

2. Place the chicken breasts (skin on, bone in) in a large bowl. Season well with pepper and salt before transferring to a sous vide bag.

3. Add fresh herbs and/or sliced lemons to the chicken bag, then vacuum seal.

4. Submerge the chicken bag into the preheated sous vide cooker. Allow it to sink and then cook until perfectly done.

Step-by-Step Instructions for Finishing the Sous Vide Cooked Chicken

1. Take the cooked chicken out of the sous vide bag. After discarding any aromatics you may have included, transfer the chicken to a plate lined with paper towels. Gently pat dry the meat on both sides to

remove excess moisture. Set aside.

2. Meanwhile, heat a skillet (cast iron) on medium-high. Add oil (vegetable/rice bran/canola), spreading evenly to coat the pan. Once the oil is shimmering hot, add the chicken, making sure its skin is facing down.

3. Cook the chicken for about two minutes or until its skin is nicely seared, crisp, and browned. Turn off the heat and let the seared chicken sit for two minutes or until slightly cooled.

4. Carefully pull out the wishbone before separating the breast meat from the breastbone.

5. Slice the chicken into four equal sized portions.

6. Serve topped with your favorite sauce, homemade vinaigrette, or lemon wedges drizzled with olive oil.

Step-by-Step Instructions for Finishing the Sous Vide Cooked Chicken Breast (Grill):

1. Take out the sous vide cooked chicken out of the bag.

Place on a plate lined with paper towels after removing any aromatics used.

2. Carefully pat the chicken with the paper towels to dry before letting it sit to cool for about two minutes or until you are finished preheating the grill.

3. Fill the chimney (half) with plenty of charcoal. Allow all charcoal to get lit before covering with gray ash and dragging the coals to the charcoal grate. Arrange the charcoal on one side before positioning the cooking grate. After covering the grill, preheat for about five minutes.

4. Making sure its skin is facing down, add the chicken to the grill and allow to cook for about four to five minutes or until crisp and brown on all sides. Transfer onto a plate and allow to cool for two minutes before removing the bones.

5. Carve the seared chicken and serve immediately.

6. Enjoy.

Recipe Using Sous Vide Cooked Chicken Breast:

Easy Chicken Salad

Ingredients:

- Lemons, whole (2 pieces)

- Parsley leaves, fresh, minced (1 tablespoon)

- Celery, diced finely (1/2 cup)

- Mayonnaise, homemade (1/4 cup + 1 tablespoon)

- Red onion, diced finely (1/2 cup)

- Dijon mustard (1 tablespoon + 1 teaspoon)

- Chives, fresh, minced (1 tablespoon)

- Salt, kosher (1/2 teaspoon)

- Black pepper, freshly ground (1/2 teaspoon)

- Tarragon sprigs, whole (4 pieces) + tarragon leaves, fresh, minced, divided (1 tablespoon)

- Garlic clove, medium, minced (1 piece)

- Chicken breast, whole, skin on, bone in, split into halves (1 ¾ pounds)

Directions:

1. Set the sous vide cooker at 150 degrees to preheat.

2. Sprinkle pepper and salt liberally on the chicken to season well. Place inside a sous vide bag and top with lemon slices (cut the 2 whole lemons into quarter-inch slices) and whole sprigs of tarragon.

3. Vacuum seal the chicken bag and place in the sous vide cooker to cook for one to four hours. Once done, transfer the chicken bag into an ice bath; set aside to chill for about fifteen minutes. (Alternatively, you can heat a large saucepot (heavy bottomed) filled with two quarts worth of water on medium-high until it reaches 155 degrees. Once the target water temperature is reached, pour the water into a cooler. Add the chicken-filled sous vide bag before sealing the cooler, then allow the chicken to cook for one to four hours, adding more boiling water as needed to keep the water temperature at 150 degrees. Once done, place the chicken bag in an ice bath and allow to chill for fifteen minutes.)

4. Combine the lemon juice (2 tablespoons) and lemon

zest (1 teaspoon) in a large bowl. Stir in the chives, minced tarragon leaves, celery, parsley, garlic, red onion, mustard, and mayonnaise. Once well-mixed, place in the refrigerator.

5. Once the sous vide cooked chicken has cooled, remove from the bag. Take out the lemon slices and tarragon stems and discard.

6. Transfer the chicken to a plate. Slice into half-inch chunks and place inside the bowl containing the mayonnaise mixture. Gently fold in the chicken chunks as you sprinkle on pepper and salt.

7. Serve your dresses sous vide chicken breast on a bed of lettuce.

8. Enjoy.

12 - Guide to Sous Vide Cooking Pulled Pork Shoulder

Step-by-Step Instructions for Sous Vide Cooking Pulled Pork Shoulder:

1. Fill the spice grinder with the mustard seed and brown sugar. Add the salt, black pepper, paprika, red pepper flakes, oregano, garlic powder, and coriander seed. Grind the ingredients until combined and reduced to a powdered mix (do this batches).

2. You might consider adding in pink curing salt (1/4 teaspoon) to the spice mixture if you prefer having a pinkish smoke ring on the pork shoulder. Reserve 3 tablespoons of your spice mix (to be used later in seasoning the meat before finishing), generously rub all over the meat to season it well.

3. Transfer the seasoned pork shoulder into a sous vide bag. Keep the seal of the sous vide bag from weakening by folding it over as you add the meat to make sure no trace of the spice mix rubs on the bag's edge. If preferred, pour in some liquid smoke (1/2 teaspoon) before vacuum sealing the bag.

4. Meanwhile, set the sous vide cooker at 165 degrees to preheat if you want your pork shoulder easy to pull apart. (If you would like your meat to be tender but sliceable, set the cooker at 145 degrees.)

5. Submerge the pork shoulder bag into the preheated water bath. Allow the meat to cook for about eighteen to twenty-four hours. Consider tenting the container with plastic wrap or aluminum foil to keep the circulator shut down due to excessive evaporation.

6. Once the sous vide pork shoulder is done, remove from the water bath. Place the pork shoulder bag in the refrigerator to chill for up to seven days if not serving right away.

7. Give the pork shoulder meat another good rub with the spice mix. This will give the meat that desired flavorful, dark, and crunchy bark after you finish it.

Step-by-Step Instructions for Finishing the Sous Vide Cooked Pulled Pork Shoulder (Smoker):

1. After lighting up the smoker, set to 300 degrees to preheat.

2. Fill with un-soaked hardwood. Once it smolders, add the sous vide cooked pork shoulder and cook for two hours and thirty minutes or until the meat can be easily pulled apart and a dark mahogany crust has developed on the surface.

Step-by-Step Instructions for Finishing the Sous Vide Cooked Pulled Pork Shoulder (Oven):

1. Set the oven to 300 degrees to preheat.

2. Place a wire rack inside a baking sheet (rimmed) lined with foil. Set the pork on the rack and place in the oven to cook for one hour and thirty minutes or until the surface develops a dark mahogany crust. Once done, take the pork shoulder out of the oven

and transfer onto a platter.

3. Use two forks or your fingers (protected by thick plastic gloves) pull the meat. Shred into chunky cuts or chop on the cutting board afterward for finer shreds.

4. Pour your favorite sauce on the pulled meat and serve right away with a soft bun and a small mound of creamy coleslaw.

Recipe Using Sous Vide Cooked Pulled Pork Shoulder:

Spicy Pulled Pork with Chorizo and Corn Slaw

Ingredients:

Pulled pork:

- Ancho chili powder (2 tablespoons)

- Black pepper, freshly ground (1/2 teaspoon)

- Cloves, ground (1/8 teaspoon)

- Garlic cloves, medium, minced (5 pieces)

- Vinegar, apple cider (2 tablespoons + 1 teaspoon)

- Cumin, ground (2 teaspoons)

- Cinnamon, ground (1/4 teaspoon)

- Oil, vegetable/ canola (2 tablespoons)

- Cornstarch (2 tablespoons)

- Yellow onion, medium, diced (1 piece)

- Amber lager, Mexican (24 ounces)

- Paprika (2 tablespoons)

- Salt, kosher (2 tablespoons)

- Coriander, ground (1/4 teaspoon)

- Pork shoulder, boneless, sliced into three-inch cubes (3 ½ pounds)

- Oregano, Mexican, dried (1 teaspoon)

- Cayenne pepper, ground (1/2 teaspoon)

- Tortillas/ burger buns (8 pieces)

Corn slaw:

- Green cabbage, shredded finely (14 ounces)

- Cotija cheese, crumbled (3 ounces)

- Honey (1 tablespoon)

- Jalapeno peppers, seeded, minced (1 piece)

- Lime juice, freshly squeezed (2 tablespoons)

- Mayonnaise, homemade (1/4 cup)

- Corn kernels, fresh cooked (2 cups)

- Garlic cloves, medium, minced (2 pieces)

- Ancho chili powder (1 tablespoon)

- Cilantro leaves, fresh, w/ intact tender stems, chopped (1/2 cup)

- Salt, kosher (1/4 teaspoon)

Directions:

1. Place all ingredients for making the corn slaw in a large bowl. Gently toss to combine, cover, and place

in the refrigerator to chill before using later.

2. Fill a medium bowl with the ground peppers as well as cloves, salt, oregano, cinnamon, paprika, cumin, coriander, and chili powder. Stir to combine and rub on all sides of the pork. Transfer the coated pork in a large bowl, cover, and place in the refrigerator to chill overnight.

3. Set the oven to 300 degrees to preheat. Meanwhile, heat a Dutch oven on medium-high before adding in the oil. Once lightly smoking, add the pork and cook (in batches) for eight minutes or until all sides are nicely browned. Once done, place the pork on a large plate.

4. Reheat the same skillet on medium. Add the onions to cook for about three minutes or until softened a bit. Stir in the garlic and cook for an additional minute.

5. Add the browned pork back to the pot. Add the beer, then allow the mixture to boil before covering and transferring to the preheated oven. Cook for about three hours or until you can easily shred the meat us-

ing two forks.

6. Once the pork is done in the oven, remove and strain (set the liquid aside in a small bowl). Transfer the pork to a large plate and shred before setting aside.

7. Meanwhile, add the reserve liquid back to the pot. Allow it to boil on medium-high before reducing heat to low and allowing it to simmer.

8. Mix water (3 tablespoons) to the cornstarch before adding to the simmering liquid in the pot. Allow the mixture to simmer for several minutes more to thicken before adding in apple cider vinegar. Add the shredded pork as well and stir to combine.

9. Place the shredded pork on warmed buns and serve with the prepared corn slaw.

13 - Guide to Sous Vide Cooking Shrimp

Step-by-Step Instructions for Sous Vide Cooking Shrimp:

1. Heat a skillet (cast iron) on low. Add olive oil (2 tablespoons) and garlic slices (2 cloves). Cook until the garlic is fragrant and tender, then stir in dried bay leaves (2 pieces) as well as smoked paprika (a pinch).

2. Once the mixture gives off a toasty paprika aroma, pour in sherry (a splash) as well as sherry vinegar (2 tablespoons). Stir to combine as you add butter (2 slices) as well.

3. Set the sous vide cooker to your target temperature to preheat.

4. Fill a sous vide bag with the shrimps. Add the flavored oil, vacuum seal, and lower into the preheated water bath. Cook for fifteen to thirty minutes or until the shrimp are plump.

5. Once done, transfer onto a platter and serve right away.

Recipe Using Sous Vide Cooked Shrimp:

Green Apple and Spicy Shrimp Salad

Ingredients:

- Water, filtered (2 quarts)

- Apples, Granny Smith, large (2 pieces)

- Cashews, plain, roasted, unsalted (1 ½ cups)

- Tomatoes, on the vine, medium (3 pieces)

- Lime juice, freshly squeezed (1 tablespoon)

- Mint leaves, fresh, torn into bits (1/3 cup)

- Shrimp, large, peeled, deveined (1 ½ pounds)

- Salt, kosher (2 tablespoons)

- Shallots, large (2 pieces) OR red onion, large (1/2 piece)

- Red pepper flakes, dried (1/4 teaspoon)

- Fish sauce, reduced sodium (1 teaspoon)

Directions:

1. Fill a large pot with water and heat on medium-high. Add salt and allow the water to boil. Once boiling, turn heat down to medium so that the boiling water is merely steaming. Use a thermometer to ensure that the water maintains a temperature between 160 and 180 degrees (the ideal temperature range needed to poach shrimp).

2. Add the shrimp to the steaming water. Stir continuously and cook for one minute or until the shrimp flesh is opaque. Once done, transfer into a colander to drain set aside in a large bowl.

3. Cut off the tops from the tomatoes before slicing them into half-inch wedged portions. Toss into the bowl containing the poached shrimp.

4. Remove the peel from the red onion, then cut into thin lengthwise slices. Toss into the shrimp bowl as well.

5. After coring the apples, slice into halves before slicing again into 1/8-inch portions. Carefully stack the apple slices and slice again to form 1/8-inch thick matchsticks, then toss into the shrimp bowl.

6. Add the red pepper flakes as well as lime juice and fish sauce. Toss gently to combine all ingredients, making sure the chicken chunks are evenly coated.

7. Toss in the mint leaves and cashews. Serve alone or with a small mound of freshly steamed rice. Enjoy.

14 - Guide to Sous Vide Cooking Halibut

Step-by-Step Instructions for Sous Vide Cooking Halibut:

1. Sprinkle generous amounts of pepper and salt on the halibut fillets (4 pieces) to season them well.

2. Place the seasoned halibut fillets inside a sous vide bag along with butter (4 teaspoons). Make sure the fillets are aligned to form a single layer. Include dill, parsley, thyme, or other aromatic herbs (you might also try adding grated citrus zest or thin shallot slices instead). Avoid putting any acidic ingredient in the bag to prevent altering the fish texture, or any chunky ingredient that may damage the fillet shapes.

3. Vacuum seal the bag to close and place in the refrigerator to rest for half an hour or overnight. This will help dry-brine and firm up the fish flesh to improve its texture and flavor.

4. Set the sous vide cooker to your target temperature.

5. Take the halibut fillets out of the refrigerator and

submerge into the water bath. Allow the fish to cook for about thirty to forty-five minutes (if you are using 1-inch-thick halibut fillets) or for forty-five minutes to one hour (if you are using 2-inch-thick halibut fillets).

6. Once the halibut fillets are done, take out of the sous vide bag and transfer onto sheets of paper towels. Take another paper towel and use to gently blot each fillet on top.

7. Remove the aromatic herbs and halibut skin to discard, then serve immediately.

8. Step-by-Step Instructions for Finishing the Sous Vide Cooked Halibut (Searing):

9. Heat a large skillet (heavy bottomed) on medium-high before adding butter (1 tablespoon). Once the butter is foaming hot, add the sous vide cooked halibut fillets and on one side for about thirty to forty-five seconds or until a bit browned.

10. Add garlic, thyme, shallots, and other aromatics to the skillet. Cook in the hot butter and use the mixture to baste the fillets. After one minute and thirty

seconds or once the halibut fillets are browned through, flip to cook on the other side for an additional fifteen to thirty seconds.

11. Drain off excess oil from the halibut fillets by placing on several sheets of paper towels. Transfer to a platter and serve.

Recipe Using Sous Vide Cooked Halibut:

Dill Halibut and Clams

Ingredients:

- Yellow onion, medium, diced (1 piece)

- White wine, dry (1 cup)

- Halibut fillets, skinless, sous vide cooked, 6-ounces (4 pieces)

- Clams, littleneck, scrubbed (12 pieces)

- Garlic cloves, medium, chopped roughly (2 pieces)

- Dill, chopped (1 tablespoon)

- Butter, unsalted, divided (4 tablespoons)

- Fennel bulb, small, halved, cored, diced (1 piece + a handful of fronds)

- Celery stalk, diced (1 piece)

- Water, filtered (2 cups)

- Salt, kosher (1/2 teaspoon)

- Black pepper, freshly ground (1/2 teaspoon)

Directions:

1. Heat a large sauté pan (straight sided) on medium-high. Add butter (2 tablespoons) and allow to melt and foam before stirring in the onion, garlic, celery, and diced fennel. Cook for about three minutes or until the vegetables are softened.

2. Pour in the wine, stir, and cook for four minutes or until the mixture is reduced to ½ its original volume. Add water as well as the sous vide cooked halibut fillets (seasoned with pepper and salt), making sure the fillets are partially submerged in cooking liquid. Surround the fillets with the clams and continue cooking until the mixture simmers. Cover and reduce heat before cooking for an additional five minutes or until

the fillets are completely cooked and the clams are open.

3. Place the halibut fillets and clams in individual bowls. Add the vegetables and set aside.

4. Meanwhile, pour broth into a pot. Add butter and dill, then whisk to combine. Once the butter is completely melted into the mixture and the broth is heated through, season with pepper and salt.

5. Pour the broth into the bowls filled with halibut and clams. Serve garnished with fennel fronds or parsley.

6. Enjoy.

15 - Guide to Sous Vide Cooking Turkey

Step-by-Step Instructions for Sous Vide Cooking Extra Crispy-Skinned Turkey Breast:

1. Take the whole turkey breast and set on a cutting board. Remove the skin, making sure to take the entire skin in one go.

2. Separate the breastbone from the breast halves by using a sharp-edged boning knife. You can set the breastbone aside for making gravy later.

3. Sprinkle liberal amounts of pepper and salt on the bottom sides of the turkey breast halves to season well.

4. Place the two turkey breast halves next to each other, ensuring that they are both aligned and matched up like jigsaw puzzle pieces. The skinny end of one breast half should be lined up next to the fatty end of the other breast.

5. Carefully press on the turkey meat to form even cyl-

indrical shapes before tying them with kitchen twine (short length) at 1" intervals. Alternating the ties on every side, begin by tying each end and then continue tying until you have reached the middle.

6. Make sure the turkey meats retain their even cylindrical shapes by adjusting with your hands.

7. Fill a sous vide bag with the tied turkey breasts. Vacuum seal and dry-brine in the refrigerator for up 3 days.

8. Set the sous vide cooker to the target temperature. Remove the dry-brined turkey from the refrigerator and place in the preheated cooker. (You can cook the turkey breasts at 145 degrees for 2 ½ hours.

9. Meanwhile, set the oven temperature at 400 degrees to preheat.

10. Use parchment paper to line a baking sheet (rimmed). Place the turkey skin on the parchment and spread to form a single layer.

11. Be generous with the pepper and salt as you season the laid-out turkey skin. Place another layer of parch-

ment paper on top and then gently press to squeeze any air pockets out.

12. Top the parchment-topped turkey skin with another baking sheet (rimmed) to help keep the turkey skin as it gets cooked.

13. Place the chicken skin in the preheated oven to cook for thirty or forty-five minutes or until really crisp. Once done, remove the skin and allow to cool down to room temperature before storing in a clean container (uncovered) for up to twenty-four hours. In case it turns soft, you can make the turkey skin crisp again by heating in the toaster oven.

14. As soon as the turkey breasts are done, remove the bags from the sous vide cooker. Take the meats out of the bags and then remove all the strings used to tie them. (You may also chill the cooked turkey breasts in the ice bath before storing in the refrigerator for one to seven days. Prior to serving, simply place the chilled turkey breast bags in the preheated water bath (set at 130 degrees) for about one hour.

15. Using even strokes, smoothly slice the turkey meats

with an extremely sharp chef's knife.

16. Place the turkey meat slices on a serving platter (warmed), making sure they form a fanned-out arrangement. Meanwhile, tear the crisp turkey skin into individual portions and place on a serving dish.

17. Serve immediately with homemade gravy and enjoy.

Recipe Using Sous Vide Cooked Extra Crispy-Skinned Turkey:

Easy Turkey Goulash

Ingredients:

- Tomatoes, stewed, diced (14 ounces)

- Tomato sauce (1 cup)

- Basil, dried (1/2 teaspoon)

- Turkey, sous vide cooked, w/ extra crispy skin, cut into one-inch chunks (1 pound)

- Garlic cloves, minced (3 pieces)

- Sugar, white (2 teaspoons)

- Pasta, bow tie (16 ounces)

Directions:

1. Heat a large skillet (nonstick) on medium.

2. Add the turkey chunks and cook until heated through.

3. Add the tomato sauce, stewed tomatoes, basil, sugar, and garlic. Stir to combine, then allow the mixture to simmer for twenty minutes. Once done, remove from heat and set aside.

4. Meanwhile, fill a large pot with water. Add salt and allow to boil. Add the bow tie pasta and cook for about eight to ten minutes or until cooked but still with a firm bite. Once done, drain and transfer into a large bowl.

5. Pour the turkey mixture onto the pasta. Gently toss to combine, making sure the pasta is evenly coated.

6. Serve right away.

16 - Guide to Sous Vide Cooking Pork Chops

Step-by-Step Instructions for Sous Vide Cooking Pork Chops:

1. Place the pork chop on a large plate. Sprinkle on generous amounts of pepper and salt to season it well.

2. Place the seasoned pork chop inside a sous vide bag and vacuum seal. Set aside while you preheat the sous vide cooker.

3. Set the sous vide cooker at 135 to 140 degrees and time for forty-five minutes to four hours of cooking. This ensures that the center will be cooked through without getting too soft.

4. Heat a skillet over medium-high. Add butter and allow it to melt and brown.

5. Once the sous vide cooked pork chop is done, remove from the bag and place it on the skillet. Cook until the meat is seared (but not burned) on all sides. Pay attention to the edges as well as the fat cap, which needs to be rendered to make it crisp and more ap-

petizing.

6. Place the seared pork chop on a plate to cool slightly for about one to two minutes.

7. Serve the seared sous vide pork chop immediately. (Alternatively, you can carve it to separate the fat cap, ribs, and loin from each other. Slice the meat into thin slices and serve right away.)

Recipe Using Sous Vide Cooked Pork Chops:

Apple Cider Pork Chops

Ingredients:

- Salt, kosher (4 tablespoons)

- Butter, unsalted, divided (4 tablespoons)

- Vinegar, apple cider (1/2 teaspoon)

- Black pepper, freshly ground (1/2 teaspoon)

- Thyme leaves, minced, divided (2 teaspoons)

- Parsley, minced (2 teaspoons)

- Pork rib chops, bone in, sous vide cooked, 1-pound (4

pieces)

- Sugar (1 tablespoon)

- Vegetable oil (2 tablespoons)

- Shallot, minced (2 tablespoons)

- Apple cider (3/4 cup)

Directions:

1. Heat a large skillet (cast iron) on medium-high before adding oil. Once heated through, add the butter (1 tablespoon) and allow to melt.

2. Stir in the thyme and shallot; cook for two minutes or until softened.

3. Pour in the apple cider. Stir to combine, reduce heat to medium, and allow the mixture to simmer for four minutes.

4. Add the cider vinegar as well as the remaining butter (3 tablespoons). Whisk well to combine before turning off the heat.

5. Sprinkle salt on the mixture and then stir in the pars-

ley.

6. Pour the prepared apple cider sauce on the sous vide pork chops.

7. Serve and enjoy.

17 - Guide to Sous Vide Cooking Tuna

Step-by-Step Instructions for Sous Vide Cooking Tuna:

1. Generously season all sides of the tuna fillets with pepper and salt.

2. Place the seasoned tuna fillets inside a large sous vide bag. Pour in some extra virgin olive (2 teaspoons for each fillet), gently turning the fillets with your hands so that all sides are evenly coated and kept from sticking to one another.

3. Include parsley/ dill/ thyme, freshly grated citrus zest, thin shallot slices, or other gentle aromatics in the tuna fillet bag. (Make sure not to add any chunky foods to avoid distorting the shape of the tuna. Avoid putting in any acidic foods as well to help retain the texture of the fish.)

4. Vacuum seal the tuna bag and place in the refrigerator overnight. This will help the tuna flesh get firmed up by the salt.

5. Meanwhile, set the sous vide cooker to the target cooking temperature to preheat as the tuna rests and gets dry-brined.

6. Submerge the tuna bag in the preheated sous vide cooker to cook for thirty to forty-five minutes (if cooking 1" thick fillets) or forty-five minutes to one hour (if cooking 2" thick fillets).

7. Once the tuna fillets are done, carefully take out of the sous vide bag and set on a large plate lined with two to three layers of paper towels. Add a layer of paper towel on top and blot gently to dry the surface of the cooked tuna fillets.

8. Remove the aromatics before placing in the refrigerator to chill.

9. Serve right away.

Step-by-Step Instructions for Finishing the Sous Vide Cooked Tuna (Stovetop):

1. Remove the aromatics before seasoning the sous vide cooked tuna fillets. You can sprinkle them with black pepper or roll them in some sesame seeds.

2. Heat a heavy skillet on high before adding oil (1 tablespoon). Allow the oil to get heated through and give off a little smoke before adding the tuna. Cook for about thirty to forty-five seconds. Flip the fish to sear on the other side, then hold sideways with tongs to sear around the edges as well.

3. Place the seared tuna on a plate lined with paper towels to drain off excess oil. Serve as is or sliced, and enjoy.

Recipe Using Sous Vide Cooked Tuna:

Tuna and Peas Orecchiette

Ingredients:

- Orechiette, dried (1 pound)

- Red chili flakes (1 teaspoon)

- Black pepper, freshly ground (1/2 teaspoon)

- Olive oil, extra virgin (1/3 cup)

- Lemon zest, freshly grated (1 tablespoon)

- Lemon juice, freshly squeezed (2 teaspoons)

- Salt, kosher (1/2 teaspoon)

- Peas, frozen (1 cup)

- Garlic clove, peeled, sliced thinly (1 piece)

- Tuna, sous vide cooked with olive oil (5 ounces)

- Parsley leaves, fresh, chopped (1/4 cup)

Directions:

1. Fill a large pot with salted water. Allow it to boil before adding the pasta; cook following the directions indicated on the package.

2. About half a minute before the pasta is al dente, stir the peas into the boiling salted water.

3. Once the pasta and peas are done, drain into a large bowl and set aside. Meanwhile, reserve some of the cooking liquid (about ½ cup).

4. Heat a small skillet over medium before adding olive oil. Once the oil shimmers, stir in the garlic as well as chili flakes. Cook for one minute or until fragrant, then place in a small bowl. Set aside.

5. Place the cooked pasta into a clean pot. Break the sous vide cooked tuna into flaked chunks and add to the pasta. Pour in the chili oil mixture before heating the pot on high.

6. Stir the pasta mixture as you add the reserved pasta liquid (1/2 cup), lemon juice and lemon zest. Continue stirring until the mixture is thickened and the pasta is evenly coated with it.

7. Serve sprinkled with pepper and salt, then topped with parsley.

8. Enjoy.

18 - Guide to Sous Vide Cooking Lobster

Step-by-Step Instructions for Sous Vide Cooking Lobster:

1. Plunge a knife straight into the heads of two live lobsters (whole, each weighing 1½ pounds). Once killed, split each lobster's carapace into halves and twist off their claws and tails.

2. After discarding the carapace, lay the lobster tails flat against a heavy cutting board. Stick 2 skewers (wooden/metal) through the tails; set aside on a large plate.

3. Fill a large pot with water and heat on high. Once boiling, add the lobster tails as well as the claw. Cook the tails for one minute before transferring to an ice bath. Once the tails are cooked after four additional minutes, transfer into the ice bath as well.

4. After shucking the lobster tails, remove the meat and place in a large bowl. Set aside.

5. Crack the shell of the lobster claws to open, then ex-

tract the meat and add to the bowl containing the meat from the lobster tails.

6. Remove the meat from the lobster knuckles and place in the same bowl containing the tail and claw meat.

7. Set the sous vide cooker to the target temperature.

8. Transfer the lobster meat into a sous vide bag. Top with unsalted butter (2 tablespoons) and fresh tarragon sprigs (2 pieces). Vacuum seal and submerge into the sous vide cooker.

9. Allow the lobster meat to cook for twenty minutes to one hour.

10. Once done, remove the bag from the cooker. Take out the lobster meat (minus the tarragon) and set on a platter. Top with hot clarified butter (1/4 cup) and lemon wedges.

11. Serve immediately.

Recipe Using Sous Vide Cooked Lobster:

Mayo Lobster Rolls

Ingredients:

- Lobster, sous vide cooked, completely cooled (2 ½ pounds)

- Mayonnaise, homemade (2 tablespoons)

- Chives, fresh, minced (1/2 tablespoon)

- Tarragon, fresh, minced (1/2 tablespoon)

- Salt, kosher (1/2 teaspoon)

- Black pepper, freshly ground (1/2 teaspoon)

- Butter, unsalted (2 tablespoons)

- Hotdog buns, top split (4 pieces)

- Rib celery, diced finely (1 piece)

- Lemon juice, freshly squeezed (1 tablespoon)

Directions:

1. Heat a large skillet over medium. Add the butter and allow to melt and foam.

2. Add the hot dog buns to the butter, making sure their exposed crumbs sides are facing down. Cook until golden brown before flipping to the other side. After

half a minute, place the hot dog buns on a platter. Set aside.

3. Take the herbs inside the sous vide bag containing the lobster. Transfer the cooked lobster to a plate and chop into one-inch cubes. Place in a large bowl.

4. Add celery, tarragon/ chives, mayonnaise, and lemon juice to the lobster bowl. Gently toss to combine, then season with pepper and salt.

5. Top the hot dog buns with the lobster mixture and serve right away.

19 - Guide to Sous Vide Cooking Carnitas

Step-by-Step Instructions for Sous Vide Cooking Carnitas:

1. Place the pork meat in a large bowl.

2. Add onion (1 piece, roughly chopped), garlic cloves (2 pieces), freshly squeezed orange juice, orange slices (from 1 fruit), bay leaves (2 pieces), and cinnamon stick (1 piece). Toss with the pork, then fold in some salt (1/2 tablespoon) to season the meat well and help it stay moist when cooked.

3. Place the seasoned pork in the sous vide bag. Add the aromatics before vacuum sealing the bag.

4. Set the sous vide cooker at your target temperature to preheat. Drop the pork meat bag into the water bath and allow it to sink. Cook until the meat is tenderly done, then remove from the cooker.

5. Take the sous vide cooked pork out of the bag and place in a large bowl. Discard the aromatics and set the bag juices aside.

6. Use forks to shred the pork meat immediately.

7. Place the shredded pork on a baking sheet (rimmed). Cook under the broiler (preheated), turning the meat occasionally until all sides are crisp and browned. (Alternatively, add the shredded meat to a skillet pre-heated on medium-high; toss in the pan until crisp on all sides. Or, if you sous vide cooked the pork meat at 145 to 165 degrees, slice into large cubes before cooking in a preheated skillet until browned and seared all over.)

Recipe Using Sous Vide Cooked Carnitas:

Salsa Verde Sous Vide Carnitas

Ingredients:

- Cinnamon stick, cut into 4 portions (1 piece)

- Onion, medium, chopped roughly (1 piece)

- Orange, medium, w/ intact peel (1 piece)

- Salt, kosher (1/2 teaspoon)

- Pork shoulder, boneless, sliced into two-inch-thick

portions (4 pounds)

- Bay leaves (2 pieces)

- Garlic cloves, medium (6 pieces)

Salsa verde:

- Anchovy fillets (6 pieces)

- Mustard (a dollop)

- Basil leaves (a handful)

- Lemon juice, freshly squeezed (1 tablespoon)

- Parsley, flat leaf (a handful)

- Capers (1 tablespoon)

- Garlic clove (1 piece)

- Olive oil, extra virgin (8 tablespoons)

Garnishings:

- Lime wedges

- Salsa verde, charred

- White onion, chopped

- Cilantro leaves, fresh

- Corn tortillas, warm

Directions:

1. Place the pork in a large bowl. Add the cinnamon stick, onion, bay leaves, and garlic.

2. Squeeze the juice out of the orange and into the pork mixture bowl. Add salt and then toss until well-combined.

3. Place the pork mixture into a sous vide bag. Vacuum seal and place in the sous vide cooker to cook to the target time and temperature.

4. Once the pork meat is done, remove from the sous vide bag and place in a large bowl. Transfer any meat chunks onto a baking sheet (rimmed) after discarding the pouch juices and aromatic herbs,

5. Roughly shred the pork meat and then spread at the bottom of the baking sheet. Set aside.

6. Place all ingredients for the salsa verde in a medium bowl. Whisk well to combine; set aside.

7. Meanwhile, set the broiler on high to preheat. Cook the pork under the broiler for about ten minutes or until crisp and nicely browned.

8. Remove the carnitas from the broiler and divide among warm tortillas. Garnish with cilantro/ white onion/ lime wedges.

9. Serve alongside the salsa verde and enjoy.

20 - Guide to Sous Vide Cooking Glazed Vegetables

Step-by-Step Instructions for Sous Vide Cooking Glazed Vegetables:

1. Set the sous vide cooker at 183 degrees to preheat.

2. Scrub one pound of whole baby carrots thoroughly before peeling. Alternatively, you can use one pound of medium or large carrots; chop into one inch cubes after scrubbing and peeling.

3. Fill a sous vide bag with the carrots. Add unsalted butter (2 tablespoons), granulated sugar (1 table-spoon), and kosher salt (1/2 teaspoon).

4. Vacuum seal the carrot bag and then submerge in the preheated water bath. Cook for one hour or until the carrots are completely tender. (If not serving right away, place in the refrigerator; use within one week.)

5. Remove the sous vide cooked carrots out of the bag and transfer onto a large skillet (heavy bottomed). Heat on high and cook, stirring frequently, for two minutes or until the liquid is reduced and glossy.

6. Sprinkle additional kosher salt (1/4 teaspoon) as well as black pepper (1/4 teaspoon) on the carrot mixture. Stir to combine. Add fresh chopped parsley (1 table-spoon) into the mix and stir again. In case the glaze breaks, you can always stir in a little water to bring back the glaze.

7. Serve right away.

8. You can easily replace the carrots, using the same steps, with any of these vegetables:

- Turnips, small, peeled, w/ trimmed stems, chopped into one-inch cubes

- Baby artichokes, trimmed, sliced into quarters

- Radishes, small, scrubbed, w/ trimmed stems

- Onions, small, peeled

- Parsnips, peeled, chopped into one-inch chunks

Recipe Using Sous Vide Cooked Glazed Vegetables:

Deliciously Glazed Carrots

Ingredients:

- Butter (1 tablespoon)

- Sugar, granulated (1/8 teaspoon)

- Nutmeg, ground (1/8 teaspoon)

- Salt, kosher (1/4 teaspoon)

- Black pepper, freshly ground (1/4 teaspoon)

- Baby carrots, Chantenay (1 pound)

- Ginger, ground (1/8 teaspoon)

- Clove, ground (1/8 teaspoon)

- Water, filtered (1/4 cup)

Directions:

1. Fill a large skillet with water.

2. Add the carrots as well as sugar, butter, nutmeg, clove, and ginger. Stir to combine.

3. Cook for about fifteen minutes or until the carrots have tenderized and the glaze has thickened.

4. Stir in pepper and salt.

5. Serve and enjoy.

21 - Guide to Sous Vide Cooking Other Favorite Foods

Step-by-Step Instructions for Sous Vide Cooking Poached Eggs:

1. Place eggs in the preheated water bath to cook to your desired level of tenderness; between 143 and 145 degrees would be great, especially if you cook the eggs for forty-five minutes. (Once the eggs are done, you may let the eggs sit at 130 degrees before serving; you might also place them in the refrigerator to rest overnight.)

2. Take the eggs out of their shells by gently hitting the large ends of the shells on a cutting board or any flat surface. Once cracked, use your right hand's fingertips to carefully remove a tiny part of the peel as you hold an entire egg with your left hand. Doing so will cause the watery egg white (loose) to start dripping out of the shell. Repeat with the rest of the eggs.

3. Place the peeled eggs in a large bowl. Do this gently so that what comes out of each shell is a smooth-edged, soft, gelled egg white with the egg yolk intact

inside. Make sure any loose egg white portions are left in the shells (you can do this by carefully spooning out the eggs prior to dumping out the loose egg white parts).

4. Meanwhile, heat a pot filled with water on medium-high and allow to boil. Once boiling, reduce heat to low and wait for the water to barely simmer. Add the peeled eggs at this point and allow them to start setting around their edges.

5. Keep the eggs from sticking to the pot as well as becoming distended to one side by swirling the simmering water from time to time. Let the eggs develop skins by cooking them for about one minute.

6. Once done, carefully spoon out the eggs from the pot. They should come out having a perfect oval shape, an opaque white color, and a delicate skin on the outside.

7. If not serving right away, transfer the poached eggs into a prepared ice bath, then place in the refrigerator to keep for one to two days.

8. Before serving, drop the poached eggs into a water bath set at 130 to 140 degrees for about ten minutes.

Step-by-Step Instructions for Sous Vide Cooking Soft-Boiled Eggs:

1. Cook the eggs as you normally would a 3-minute egg: Heat a pot filled with water until boiling; carefully drop in the eggs and let them sit for three minutes, and transfer them into an ice bath.

2. Meanwhile, set the sous vide cooker at 143 degrees to preheat.

3. After one minute in the ice bath, remove the eggs and submerge in the preheated water bath. Allow them to cook for forty-five minutes.

4. Peel the sous vide soft-boiled eggs as you would a regular soft-boiled egg.

Step-by-Step Instructions for Sous Vide Cooking Bacon:

1. Set the sous vide cooker at 145 degrees.

2. Fill a sous vide bag with the bacon (1 pound, thick-cut) OR leave the bacon in its original plastic container. Submerge in the sous vide cooker to cook for eight to forty-eight hours.

3. Once done, take the bacon out of the water bath and place in the refrigerator to chill, store in the freezer for using later, or serve immediately.

4. Finish your sous vide bacon by first heating a large skillet for five minutes on medium-high. Add the bacon and let cook on one side for two minutes or until crisp and browned. Flip the bacon to cook on the other side for about fifteen seconds or until no longer pale.

5. Place the bacon pieces on a plate lined with paper towels. Allow any excess fat drain off before serving.

Step-by-Step Instructions for Sous Vide Cooking Breakfast Ham:

1. Set the sous vide cooker at 145 degrees to preheat.

2. Meanwhile, fill a sous vide bag with breakfast ham (8

slices, stacked/separated).

3. Drop the ham-filled bag into the preheated water bath. Cook for six to twelve hours.

4. Once the sous vide ham is done, place in the refrigerator and use within one week, store in the freezer and use within three months (before finishing and serving, thaw in the refrigerator overnight first), or serve right away.

Heat a large skillet (cast iron/ stainless steel) on medium-high. Add vegetable oil (1 tablespoon) and allow to shimmer and get heated through. Add the sous vide ham and cook for about two minutes or until crisp and nicely seared on just one side. Place on a warm platter, serve and enjoy.

Thank You

As we reach the end of this book, I want to say thanks for reading this book.

I want to get this information out to as many people as possible. If you found this book helpful, I would greatly appreciate you leaving me a review. This helps others find the book as well.

Disclaimer

This document is geared towards providing exact and reliable information in regards to the topic and issue covered. The publication is sold on the idea that the publisher is not required to render an accounting, officially permitted, or otherwise, qualified services. If advice is necessary, legal, financial, medical or professional, a practiced individual in the profession should be ordered.

This information is not presented by a financial or medical practitioner and is for entertainment, educational and informational purposes only. The content is not intended as a substitute for professional medical advice, diagnosis, or treatment. Always seek the advice of your physician or other qualified health care provider with any questions you may have regarding a medical condition. Never disregard professional medical advice or delay in seeking it because of something you have read.

The information provided herein is stated to be truthful and consistent, in that any liability, in terms of inattention or otherwise, by any usage or abuse of any policies, processes, or directions contained within is the solitary and utter responsibility of the recipient reader. Under no circumstances will any legal responsibility or blame be held against the

DISCLAIMER

publisher for any reparation, damages, or monetary loss due to the information herein, either directly or indirectly.

Last Updated: 11.Dec.2017